THE
PROSTATE CANCER
ANSWER BOOK

Other Avon Books by
Marion Morra and Eve Potts

CHOICES

TRIUMPH:
GETTING BACK TO NORMAL
WHEN YOU HAVE CANCER

THE PROSTATE CANCER ANSWER BOOK

AN UNBIASED GUIDE TO TREATMENT CHOICES

MARION MORRA & EVE POTTS

Illustrations by Hilda R. Muinos

AVON BOOKS 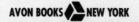 NEW YORK

This book was current to the best of the authors' knowledge at publication, but before acting on information herein, the consumer should, of course, verify the information with an appropriate physician or agency. NOTE: The designations that treatments are standard or under clinical evaluation are not to be used as a basis for reimbursement determinations.

THE PROSTATE CANCER ANSWER BOOK is an original publication of Avon Books. This work has never before appeared in book form.

AVON BOOKS
A division of
The Hearst Corporation
1350 Avenue of the Americas
New York, New York 10019

Copyright © 1996 by Marion Morra and Eve Potts
Illustrations copyright © 1996 by Hilda R. Muinos
Published by arrangement with the authors
Library of Congress Catalog Card Number: 96-5684
ISBN: 0-380-78564-1

Library of Congress Cataloging in Publication Data:
Morra, Marion E.
    The prostate cancer answer book : an unbiased guide to treatment
    choices / Marion Morra and Eve Potts.
        p.   cm.
Includes bibliographical references and index.
1. Prostate—Cancer—Popular works.   I. Potts, Eve.   II. Title.
RC280.P7M67   1996   95-5684
616.99'463—dc20   CIP

First Avon Books Trade Printing: September 1996

AVON TRADEMARK REG. U.S. PAT. OFF. AND IN OTHER COUNTRIES, MARCA REGISTRADA, HECHO EN U.S.A.

Printed in the U.S.A.

OPM   10 9 8 7 6 5 4 3 2 1

Dedicated to Robert A. Potts
who inspired us to get the facts on prostate cancer
after he was diagnosed with it fifteen years ago.
His insistence on understanding the choices
and his determination
not to be pushed into a radical procedure
made us aware of how much treatment
of males with prostate cancer
parallels what happened in past decades
to women with breast cancer.
We salute his good sense and his good health!

Foreword
by Dr. V. T. DeVita, Jr.

One of the most pressing questions in medicine today is how to manage prostate cancer. Lots of things are happening, most of them good, that are changing how prostate cancer is understood and treated. It is one of the most common cancers in men, with a skyrocketing incidence. Like breast cancer, however, the mortality rate from the disease is nowhere near its incidence. That is, many more people are diagnosed with the disease than die from it. That usually means one of two things: either you're doing something right in regard to diagnosis and treatment or the cancers being diagnosed are not life threatening. We, as physicians, don't know which is true for prostate cancer at the present time.

The availability of the PSA test in the early 1980s offered a tool we thought would tell us which cancers in the prostate might be serious enough to treat, but it will take much more time to determine whether this is true or not. Are there cases that do not need to be treated? If not, why screen for the disease with the PSA test and create the burden of "knowing" a tumor is present if it means little? The whys and wherefores of the PSA test are central to all these questions and are well covered in this book. If we are to treat the disease, how do we treat it? Surgeons favor surgery; radiotherapists favor radiotherapy.

The standard methods of treatment were all also refined at the same time the PSA test came along. It became possible to deliver radiation treatment more accurately. A technique was perfected for surgery that could spare important nerves in the region of the prostate. Both improvements reduced side effects somewhat and inspired their advocates. In addition, new hormones and drugs have come upon the scene. The good news is that the dilemmas of which to treat and how to treat usually occur at a time in a

disease when there is lots of new information on management—
a sign of better things to come. Until this happens, the bad news
is we must make do with some confusion.

It is difficult for the public to understand how doctors can dis-
agree on things like this, but we do, and our conflicts are often
colored by the biases we acquire in the long period of training it
takes to become a doctor and to specialize, so they can be com-
pounded by which physician you happen to see first. We are also
often called upon these days to air our differences via the media.
People who are well often tune this out, but for someone diagnosed with prostate cancer, this can create a lot of added confusion.

So what do you do in a situation like this? Read this book! It is
a neutral and dispassionate review of the available information in
a format that is easy for laypeople to understand. I found it re-
markably readable, which didn't surprise me, since it was written
by two women who have coauthored a number of other prize-
winning books that have served to guide patients through the
complexity of cancer and all of its ramifications.

This well-researched book also presents all the modern approaches to the treatment of prostate cancer. As the authors
stress, a man has time to make a careful treatment choice with
prostate cancer. Armed with the kind of information in this book,
men are in a much better position to ask doctors appropriate
questions and know when the answers make sense and, ultimately,
to make informed decisions. The details on the potential side
effects of each treatment are particularly well handled. This is
important, because it is around the discussion of side effects that
a treatment decision is often made. This is not always handled
well by doctors, who tend more often than not to believe that the
disease is always worse than the cure. In prostate cancer, this is
often not the case.

Experts like these authors, who are not laden with the burden
of being physicians or with the disease itself, are a good source
of information. These two authors have acquired their expertise
through a long association with the National Cancer Institute and
the Yale Cancer Center, as well as with the American Cancer Society, and through developing books and systems to foster better
communication between the public and the medical profession.

It may seem curious that two women who run no risk of developing the disease should serve as advocates for a more reasoned management of prostate cancer. But not too many men—save for a few physicians—have stepped up to the issue so far, so I say more power to the authors. There may be doctors who will feel threatened by this and by the expert simplification of a truly complex subject, but patients who read the book won't mind.

Vincent T. DeVita, Jr., MD,
Director, Yale Cancer Center

Dr. DeVita was appointed the Director of the National Cancer Institute by the President of the United States in 1980 and served until 1988, when he became Physician-in-Chief at Memorial Sloan-Kettering Cancer Center, in New York City.

Acknowledgments

This book bears our names on its cover, but the real authors number in the thousands, starting with Eve's husband who, 15 years ago, was faced with the need for information in making important decisions about his treatment for prostate cancer. Much of the information is drawn from the experiences of hundreds of men who, like Bob, endured treatments and shared with us what they would have liked to have known before starting on the cancer journey. From the start, they and their families led us by sharing their everyday experiences and problems in dealing with prostate cancer. We have been enlightened and enriched by these encounters and by the willingness of these men to talk frankly with us about their concerns, dilemmas, and questions.

In sifting through information for this book, we have dealt with countless documents and research reports, scribbled notes at ocology seminars and workshops, absorbed information from original scientific writings and medical textbooks, and had face-to-face discussions with dozens of doctors. The materials from the National Cancer Institute, especially the state-of-the-art statements and the American Cancer Society's textbooks and research reports, were of inestimable value.

We tried, as we have in our numerous editions of *Choices*, to make this a book written from the point of view of the person who has cancer. Because the terminology is that used in hospitals and doctors' offices, we tried to clarify the language throughout the book so that when it is encountered during treatment, it will be understandable. We have defined the terms so that in discussions with members of the medical profession, who use these words, some of them real tongue twisters, in talking with you about your condition, you will be on familiar territory. We hope this book will make it possible for you to ask more detailed ques-

xiiACKNOWLEDGMENTS

tions and therefore enter into more meaningful discussions, helping you to become a partner with your doctor in dealing with
your cancer.

A group of professionals in the cancer field helped us to avoid
medical pitfalls in our writing, answered and clarified our many
questions and reviewed our material in their areas of expertise.
Among them were: Dr. Vincent T. DeVita, MD, Director of the
Yale Cancer Center; Dr. Joseph Cardinale, MD, Assistant Director,
Department of Radiation Oncology, Hospital of St. Raphael, New
Haven; Dr. Bernard Litton, MD, Professor of Surgery (Urology),
Yale University Medical Center; Dr. John P. Long, MD, Depart-
ment of Urology (Cryosurgery), New England Medical Center
Hospitals, Boston; and Frank Vanoni, MD, Family Practitioner,
Charlotte Hungerford Hospital, Torrington, Connecticut. We also
owe a special debt of gratitude to Bob Potts, Roy Dickinson, Tom
Murphy, John Moran, Al Crosby, and Grant Scott, who were es-
pecially insightful.

Though it is through the help of many, many people that this
book came to life, we alone take responsibility for any errors or
misinterpretations.

Although this book cannot make decisions for you, we hope it
will serve you as a major resource. We have tried to interpret the
current information and controversies based on the latest knowledge in the field so that your decision will be an informed one.
The conclusions you reach will be your own, made with the help
of your doctors who know the details of your cancer.

Contents

THE

PROSTATE CANCER

ANSWER BOOK

chapter 1

Do I Need to Do Something If My PSA Is Not Normal?

Many men, after getting a diagnosis of a high PSA (prostate-specific antigen), immediately decide that the only solution is to have a total prostatectomy. They want the cancer out. But it's not as straighforward as that. First of all, the PSA test is not the simple definitive test it is sometimes advertised to be. You need to fully understand the ramifications of your PSA test, the nature of prostate cancer, as well as the consequences of each treatment before making any decisions.

Your PSA is not normal.

You've heard all the controversies about the blood test for detecting prostate cancer early, prostate specific antigen (PSA), but you haven't paid too much attention. Now, you need some facts, because it's happened to you.

You have no symptoms, no urinary difficulties, no warnings. You went for a routine check and were told you have an abnormal PSA. That verdict opens the possibility that you may have cancer.

You are going to be faced with making some very critical medical decisions. The best advice we can give is:

- **Don't be in a hurry to make a decision.**
- **Don't do anything until you understand what your PSA reading is all about, what the implications are of possible treatments, and what other alternatives you might consider. Learn about all your choices.**
- **Remember that some decisions are irreversible.**

You've probably been raised to believe that when it comes to health the doctor knows best. Taking matters into your own hands may violate everything you've been taught. However, it's important in the case of a prostate cancer diagnosis that you study the whole picture and make a decision based on the real facts (rather than the scare of the word *cancer*) as well as on your own beliefs and lifestyle. Do your homework and get comfortable with all the possibilities and pros and cons before you decide.

During the past few years, a dramatic evolution in the detection of prostate cancer has occurred because of the use of the PSA test and ultrasound techniques. That's the good news.

The bad news is that in many cases, even when these techniques are used in a competent manner, doctors are still unable to distinguish individual patients whose cancers will not progress from those whose cancers will eventually grow and spread. Furthermore, it is no secret that top experts still cannot agree on what is the best and most effective treatment for prostate cancer.

The ramifications of the PSA blood test can take you on a roller-coaster ride of decisions that can drastically change your way of life. The possible aftereffects of the various courses of treatment available are not always clear to most men. There are many ifs, ands, and buts that you need to look into and weigh very carefully before you decide on what is right for you.

With new techniques available for detection and treatment, men have more choices than ever before. This means that decision making is very difficult. Gathering information, studying and digesting the facts, and talking with doctors from different disciplines are important, intelligent, and essential steps to take before making a decision. Treat this information gathering the way you

FACTS TO WEIGH BEFORE DECIDING YOUR NEXT STEP

FACT	YOU NEED TO KNOW
Autopsy studies show that 30–50% of all men over 50 have cancerous cells in their prostates. Many cannot be detected by the PSA test.	Many prostate cancers, because they grow very slowly, cause no problems for a long time, if ever.
Nearly 317,000 new cases of prostate cancer will be diagnosed this year.	Many of these cancers have been found through the PSA test. Over 60% of them will be diagnosed in early stages.
One study has shown excellent survival results in men, regardless of age, who have received no treatment. The study has followed these men, who have well-differentiated or moderately well-differentiated prostate cancer that is confined to the prostate, for up to 15 years. A similar study that has followed men for 4–9 years shows comparable results.	You need to decide whether or not you wish to have surgery or some other kind of treatment. More studies are showing there may be little difference in survival among the treatments. However, since much of the data that are being used are not comparable, it is difficult to decide on the right treatment.
In men over 80, autopsies show that nearly every man has some form of prostate cancer.	The longer a man lives, the greater his chance of developing prostate cancer. But only 2.9% of men die from prostate cancer.

treat buying a new car—check out all the options before you make a decision.

Do all prostate cancers need to be removed?

Because they grow very slowly, many prostate cancers cause no problems for a very long time—if ever. According to autopsy studies, 30 to 50 percent of all men over 50 have cancerous cells in their prostates. This is true even though just 2.9 percent of men die from prostate cancer. This means that there are millions of men who have cancerous cells in their prostates but never even know it.

How many men in the United States have prostate cancer?

Some 317,000 new cases of prostate cancer are being diagnosed this year, with about 60 percent of them in early stages. About 41,000 men will die as a result of prostate cancer this year.

What is my risk of having prostate cancer that requires treatment?

Doctors are making decisions about how to treat the 11 million men in the United States who have prostate cancer. That's about 40 percent of men over 50. According to one study, most of these men—about 80 percent, or nearly 9 million—will not be affected by their prostate cancer. Of the 20 percent who will be affected, half could benefit from some kind of treatment, whereas the other half will have tumors that have already spread. The problem for you and your doctor is to sort out which of these three groups you are in.

Has the number of prostate operations increased?

Between 1984 and 1990, the rate of radical prostatectomies increased by a staggering 575 percent. In 1990, more radical prostatectomies were performed on Medicare patients than were performed in 1984, 1985, and 1986 combined. And the number of radical prostatectomies performed continue to increase. Between 1991 and 1993, the number of radical prostatectomies soared from 50,000 to about 100,000. These numbers do not mean that more men are getting cancer of the prostate. What they mean is that more cancers are being found. Most of the increase is due to the PSA test, which has allowed doctors to find early indications of prostate cancer. Death rates are rising much more slowly than the number of diagnosed cases. Some of the increase in death is due to the fact that men are living longer.

How much does prostate cancer surgery extend life?

Some studies show that men who had surgery, on average, lived **only two to six months** longer than those who did not have surgery. There is some evidence that less drastic treatment—such as, in some cases, watchful waiting with frequent checkups—may be a reasonable alternative for men who are found to have localized prostate cancers. However, since there has never been a controlled trial that has compared the major treatments for early-stage cancer—surgery, radiation therapy, and watchful waiting—

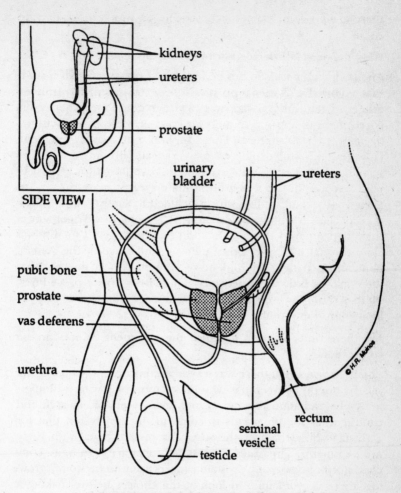

SIDE VIEW

kidneys
ureters
prostate

urinary
bladder
ureters
pubic bone
prostate
vas deferens
urethra
rectum
seminal
vesicle
testicle

© H.R. Munos

**The relationship of the prostate gland
to the other organs in the area.**

there are no comparable data available on which to make a decision.

What happens if I decide not to have treatment?

An eye-opening statistic can be found in a five-year Swedish study that followed 223 men who received no treatment for prostate cancer. Their survival rate was 92.8 percent. Researchers compared them to a group of men who had prostate cancer and underwent radical surgery. Their survival rate was 90 percent. However, this study followed men for only five years. Most researchers feel that the patients need to be followed for at least 10 years because of the slow-growing nature of prostate cancer. An analysis of several studies, which included 828 men with localized prostate cancer who had no treatment, showed that 87 percent of them had survived 10 years. In addition, their overall survival was close to what was expected of men of similar age in the general population. With more and more emerging facts showing that there may be little life expectancy gained from drastic procedures, there is cause for every man faced with a decision to take a closer look at all the options.

Are there other cancers in which the treatment choices are so controversial?

About 15 years ago, there was a similar controversy in breast cancer treatment: between having a mastectomy or having a lumpectomy plus radiation therapy. It took many years of research and clinical trials for physicians to come to the conclusion that for early-stage breast cancer the survival rates are equal with these two treatments. The issues in prostate cancer are even more complex. But because many prostate cancers seem to be slower growing, there is more time to look at the choices before making a decision.

Does a normal PSA guarantee I don't have cancer?

A normal PSA level is no guarantee that cancer is **not** there. It is possible that as many as 40 percent of men with prostate cancer have normal PSA levels. And even if the PSA does represent prostate cancer, there is no way of knowing whether testing and treatment will change the outcome or improve health in the final analysis.

EIGHT THINGS TO DO
BEFORE DECIDING ON TREATMENT

1. Ask the doctor to discuss all the possible alternatives with you.

2. Call the Cancer Information Service, toll-free, at 1-800-4-CANCER for the latest up-to-date information and facts on your type of cancer. Making this call is one of the most important things you can do for yourself. Trained personnel can talk to you about your kind of cancer and help you decide what steps to take. They also will be happy to supply you with booklets, clinical trials that are being done on your type of cancer, and Protocol Data Query (PDQ) statements from the National Cancer Institute that give you the latest information on treatments. If you have further questions at a later date, don't hesitate to call again.

3. If a medical library is available to you, look there for information. The Cancer Information Service is a good starting point for information, but you and your friends and family may want to do other research as well. So much new research is being done in so many places that you may find an important clue to a treatment that may be helpful to you.

4. Meanwhile, make sure you have the right doctor. The kind of treatment you get depends on how much your doctor knows about your particular kind of cancer. Ask your doctor about clinical trials and the latest PDQ statement from the National Cancer Institute on your kind of cancer.

5. There are doctors (called oncologists) who specialize in treating cancer. Beyond that there are specialists in every kind of cancer, down to specialists who deal exclusively with one cell type of cancer. Get an opinion on treatment from someone who is treating your type of disease on a daily basis.

(continued)

EIGHT THINGS TO DO
BEFORE DECIDING ON TREATMENT *(cont.)*

6. If during your research you find a doctor who has written a paper on your type of cancer, don't hesitate to call and discuss your case.

7. If at all possible, a second opinion should be sought at the start before submitting to any cancer treatment of any kind. The original diagnosis and treatment plan you were given will probably be confirmed, but you deserve the right to have your doctor's diagnosis confirmed and any other possible treatments explored and explained to you. Take the time to do your homework. A few extra weeks usually will not make any difference as far as the progress of the cancer is concerned but can make all the difference in your future.

8. In many cases, a second pathological opinion is a good idea. The pathology report is the basis on which all future decisions will be made, and although some cancers are pathologically diagnosed without any question, you need to check to make certain this is the case for you.

Are symptoms of cancer similar to those of other prostate problems?

Most patients with early prostate cancer have no symptoms. However, three out of four men over age 50 have some symptoms of an enlarged prostate, which in most cases are not due to cancer (see Chapter 3).

chapter 2

What Does the PSA Test Really Mean?

> The greatest danger of the prostate-specific antigen (PSA) test is the risk that it will trigger unnecessary treatment. That's why it's important to monitor what is happening to you and not to panic when you are faced with an elevated PSA.

On average, normal PSA levels range from 0 to 4 nanograms per milliliter (ng/ml). When a PSA level is from 4 to 10 ng/ml, it is considered to be moderately elevated. Levels over 10 ng/ml are considered high. However, you shouldn't jump to conclusions if your PSA is beyond these ranges. Many factors are involved, such as prostate enlargement, inflammation, infection, age, family background, as well as some unknowns and unexplainables. Physicians and researchers are continuing to reevaluate these PSA values as more data become available.

FACTS TO REMEMBER ABOUT PSA

- You can have an elevated PSA reading because of a nonmalignant enlargement called *benign prostatic hyperplasia* (BPH).

9

- Prostatitis caused by an inflammation or infection of the prostate can elevate your PSA.
- If you have a large prostate, your PSA can be elevated because PSA is made by both benign and cancerous cells.
- Recent findings show that PSA levels increase significantly after ejaculation and remain elevated for at least six hours, usually returning to normal after 48 hours. To get an accurate PSA reading, it is recommended that you abstain from ejaculation for 48 hours before getting a PSA test.
- PSA values may fluctuate by as much as 30 percent for physical reasons.
- Even though the substance measured by the PSA test is made by both cancerous and noncancerous cells, cancerous prostates make about 10 times as much of the substance as benign prostates.
- New studies indicate that total PSA is composed of free and complexed molecules. Complexed molecules appear to be associated with cancer. It is possible for urologists to determine the ratio of free PSA molecules to total PSA. One study indicates that if the ratio is more than 0.15 the probability of cancer is very low and you probably do not need a biopsy. If your ratio is 0.15 or less, you should proceed with a biopsy since there is indication that you have a high ratio of complexed molecules.
- If your PSA reading is between 4 and 10, there is only about a 20 percent chance of your having prostate cancer.
- On the other hand, a PSA reading of under 4 does not guarantee that you do not have cancer. Sometimes a small cancer does not make enough PSA to raise the reading. (In very rare cases, a very malignant cancer might be of such a primitive form that it is unable to make any PSA.)
- Even with very high PSA levels, there is the possibility that the cancer is confined to the prostate gland.
- A steadily rising PSA is more indicative of cancer than a one-time reading. It is the average consistent increase in the PSA reading over months or years that is more significant than a single reading.
- The PSA test is also used in tracking what is happening to a man who has prostate cancer.

What is the PSA test?

The PSA test is a blood test that measures prostate-specific antigen, a protein produced by the prostate gland. First approved in 1986, the PSA test was used to monitor prostate cancer patients' response to treatments. Its success led to its use as a screening tool. The American Cancer Society recommended its use as a routine screening test in 1992. Since it came into play as a screening device, the number of prostate cancers being discovered has increased enormously—from 134,000 in 1992 to 317,000 in 1996. The National Cancer Institute (NCI) states that the PSA, a test developed with NCI funding, is a potentially promising screening test. However, there is insufficient evidence on which to decide its effectiveness as a routine screening test in men who do not have prostate cancer. The NCI is presently conducting a trial to test the value of early detection with the PSA and with the digital rectal exam on reducing deaths from prostate cancer.

Has the number of men who have prostate cancer increased recently?

Prostate cancer cases have risen an average of 3.9 percent annually since 1973. From 1987 until 1991, the increase was 12.1 percent. The median age of diagnosis is 72. Prostate cancer rates are 37 percent higher for black men than for white men.

Why has there been such a dramatic increase in the number of prostate cancer cases?

Much, if not all, of the increase is believed to come from new tests and procedures being used, especially the wide availability of the PSA test, rather than an increase in the actual number of prostate cancers. Even before the PSA test was available, the use of the surgical procedure known as transurethral resection of the prostate (TURP), commonly used in the late 1970s and 1980s, revealed many cases of latent prostate cancer. A hospital-based survey by the American College of Surgeons reported that 68.4 percent of prostate cancer patients diagnosed in 1990 had been tested for PSA, compared with only 5.8 percent in 1984.

How many of the men who have prostate cancer die as a result of it?

The number of deaths per year has been rising slowly, but much more slowly than the number of newly diagnosed cases. Deaths have risen about 1 percent per year from 1973 to 1991. From 1987 to 1991, the annual rate of increase was 2.9 percent. Death rates have increased most in men aged 85 and older. It is believed that the large number of men who are living to be over 85 may be contributing to the increase in prostate cancer deaths.

What does the PSA test tell the doctor?

The PSA is a protein measured in the blood that is produced by both normal and malignant prostate cells. The level can be elevated above the normal range if there is pronounced inflammation or if there is a sudden blockage of blood supply to a portion of the prostate gland. The PSA test alone, however, cannot tell you with absolute certainty whether or not you have prostate cancer. It must be used with other indicators to determine diagnosis. The PSA readings for both cancer and other diseases of the prostate can range from zero up into the hundreds.

How much do PSA values vary?

There are no uniform standards for PSA tests. Establishing a normal range for the PSA value has been difficult. Cancer has been discovered in patients with ranges from 0.2 to over 150 ng/ml. Thirty-six percent of patients with nonmalignant tumors have a moderately elevated PSA. An abnormally high PSA level, however, may suggest cancer of the prostate. When PSA levels continue to rise progressively higher over a period of time, further testing is indicated. It is important to have subsequent PSA tests processed by the same laboratory because there are several manufacturers of the test, each of which reports results differently. Even if the same laboratory changes to a different PSA test, the results may not be comparable.

What are considered to be normal PSA levels?

Researchers are continuing to study this question. It appears that
normal levels may differ according to age. Recent studies suggest
the following age-specific PSA levels:

- Age 71–80: 6.5 ng/ml
- Age 61–70: 4.5 ng/ml
- Age 51–60: 3.5 ng/ml
- Age 41–50: 2.4 ng/ml

In addition, an annual rise in PSA level of about 0.04 ng/ml in
men over age 60 is not considered abnormal. For men over 70, a
6.5 is considered a normal level. These continuing studies will
suggest changes in both the guidelines and in follow-up practices.
As a general rule, a PSA level that is higher than 10 to 15 ng/ml
in the absence of other findings is highly suggestive of prostate
cancer. **Higher PSA readings have been recorded in men who
have enlarged prostates, have just undergone a transurethral resection of the prostate (TURP), who ejaculated 48 hours before
the PSA blood was drawn, or who have a serious infection.**

WHAT THE PSA LEVELS MEAN	
0–4 ng/ml	Considered normal level; can vary by age:
• 2.4 ng/ml	Considered normal for ages 41–50
• 3.5 ng/ml	Considered normal for ages 51–60
• 4.5 ng/ml	Considered normal for ages 61–70
• 6.5 ng/ml	Considered normal for ages 71–80
4–10 ng/ml	Moderately elevated
Over 10 ng/ml	High

What factors other than cancer can cause the PSA to rise?

The most common reason for the false-positive result of a PSA
reading is an enlarged prostate. Because an enlarged prostate produces benign prostatic tissue, it produces more PSA. It is also
known that if you have prostatitis, your PSA level rises temporarily.

A major trauma or injury to your prostate, such as an operation or a biopsy, can kick up your PSA level 50-fold for about two weeks.

REASONS WHY YOUR PSA MAY BE HIGH

- Enlarged prostate.
- Infection or stones in your prostate.
- Infection in your urinary tract.
- Surgery on your prostate (such as TURP).
- Ejaculation within 48 hours of test.
- Biopsy on your prostate.
- Prostate cancer.

Can a man who doesn't have cancer have a high PSA?

The rise in PSA is sometimes seen in men who do not have cancer, and occasionally there may be normal PSA readings in men who **do** have cancer of the prostate. The size and weight of the prostate is a factor in making a judgment. **Nonetheless, the PSA does serve as an indicator, and when it is found to be beyond the normal range, further testing is important to determine if the cause is cancer.**

If I have an infection, will my PSA go back to normal immediately?

It usually takes the PSA several weeks to get back to normal after the infection has been treated and resolved. Your doctor will probably check your PSA a couple of months after your infection has completely cleared up.

Are there other values of the PSA that might have significance in a diagnosis?

Some urologists consider the density of the PSA to be helpful in making a diagnosis. On the other hand, other physicians feel that this test is not very reliable. When an ultrasound examination of the prostate is done, it is possible to determine the size, in cubic centimeters, and the weight, in grams, of the entire prostate. The PSA density is then calculated by dividing the PSA value by the weight of the prostate. If the number resulting from this is 0.15

(nanograms per milliliter per cubic centimeter of prostate size) or less, many believe that this is an indication that cancer is probably not present. If the density is 0.2 or higher, there is a greater chance that cancer may be present.

Where does the doctor get the blood for the PSA test?

Most men are not even aware they are giving blood for a PSA test because it is often part of routine testing. It is usually requested by the doctor along with blood cholesterol and other blood tests that are routinely done during physicals or it may be automatically included by the laboratory along with the standard battery of tests run on a blood sample.

How long does it take to get the results of my PSA test?

It depends on the laboratory, the time of the week you are having the test done, and the lab's work schedule. The results usually come back to your doctor within a couple of days. Make sure you ask your doctor when and how you will be given the results. Also, if you wish to have your own copy of the results of your tests, be sure to request it when you are having the tests done. Some men who have prostate cancer like to keep track and monitor their own test results and keep a notebook with all the information involving their treatments.

PSA RECORD
Date   PSA Reading

Keeping a record of your PSA is simple. Just use one page of your medical notebook to record your PSA readings.

Does the digital rectal exam affect the PSA level?

The digital exam has no significant effect on PSA levels. Many doctors, however, try to do this test **after** blood has been taken for PSA testing.

Is the PSA test a substitute for the digital rectal exam?

No. Many men wish they could skip the digital rectal exam and just have what seems to be the simpler blood test. However, used alone, the PSA test does not diagnose prostate cancer. It is im-

> Important note: PSA blood tests should be done before cystoscopy or needle biopsy because these procedures may raise the PSA levels. The digital exam by itself does not significantly increase serum PSA, but cystoscopy and needle biopsy may. PSA levels can increase after ejaculation, returning to normal within 48 hours.

portant to have the digital rectal exam because it gives the doctor the chance to feel whether or not there are lumps that can be felt.

What other blood studies are usually done to check for prostate cancer?

In addition to the PSA test, a prostatic acid phosphatase (PAP) test may be done. The prostatic fraction of serum acid phosphatase is made by the normal cells in the prostate gland, but it is also made in equal amounts by any cancerous cells that may be within the prostate. Cancerous cells may escape the prostate and appear in other parts of the body, where they continue to make acid phosphatase, elevating the levels. The values are usually normal when there is no cancer in the prostate or when the cancer is confined to the prostate.

What is a PAP test and what does it indicate?

The level of PAP rises above normal in many prostate cancer patients especially if the cancer has spread beyond the prostate. This test gives the doctor one more possible clue to use in determining how to proceed. There are a number of other conditions that can raise the PAP level—BPH, prostatitis, Paget's disease, pneumonia, and hepatitis. The drug Atromid-S, which is taken to lower cholesterol levels, can raise the PAP level. A rectal exam to check the prostate may also raise the PAP level. The PSA has taken the place of the PAP test for screening for early prostate cancer.

What happens to the PSA after treatment?

- After a successful radical prostatectomy, the PSA is expected to decline to undetectable levels—less than 0.1 ng/ml.

- After radiation treatment, the response of the PSA is slower to decline, usually not reaching a stable figure until 6 to 12 months after treatment.
- After hormone therapy, an 80 percent decline in the PSA is usually seen within the first month.

What are the usual symptoms of cancer of the prostate?

Very often there are no symptoms. However, symptoms that should not be ignored—especially if they come on suddenly—include a weak or interrupted flow of urine, an inability to urinate or difficulty in starting urination, the need to urinate frequently (especially at night), blood in the urine, urine flow that is not easily stopped, painful or burning urination, and continuous pain in the back, pelvis, or hips. These symptoms are often the same symptoms that indicate other prostate problems, but they are symptoms that should be checked by a doctor who can detect the difference between a cancerous and noncancerous enlargement of the prostate. Be aware, however, that early prostate cancer often does not cause any symptoms, which is why PSA tests and regular digital exams are often ordered.

Are there any new prostate tests that might give more definitive information?

Dr. William J. Catalona of the Washington University School of Medicine in St. Louis, who pioneered PSA testing for prostate cancer, has been perfecting a new test that could eliminate up to 75 percent of unnecessary biopsies while effectively screening for prostate cancer. The new test could help doctors distinguish between prostate cancer and BPH by isolating unbound PSA. Men with prostate cancer appear to have significantly lower levels of unbound PSA than those who do not have cancer. The proposed new test (which is not presently available but may be available shortly) will detect cancer in men with only slightly elevated PSA levels. It would eliminate many uncomfortable biopsies and save the cost of those biopsies (presently ranging in cost from $1,000 to $2,000).

chapter 3

Understanding Your Prostate and the Nature of Prostate Cancer

The prostate is a very complicated gland. Most symptoms of early prostate cancer are the same symptoms that are caused by other problems. There are no symptoms that can be said to point without question to cancer of the prostate. Because of this, it is important to have any urinary symptoms, erection problems, or back pain checked out by your doctor.

WHAT YOU NEED TO KNOW ABOUT YOUR PROSTATE

- Prostate problems don't always mean prostate cancer.
- Most men have at least one bout of prostatitis (inflammation of the prostate) in their lifetimes.
- Men who have acute prostatitis have an abrupt onset of fever, pain at the base of the penis, and painful urination.
- With chronic prostatitis you may have low-grade, recurring infections that cause discomfort. Bacterial and nonbacterial forms of chronic prostatitis require different treatments.
- The prostate also becomes enlarged as the result of hor-

monal changes associated with aging. This condition is known as benign prostatic hyperplasia (BPH). By the age of 60, prostate enlargement is found in almost all men. When this happens, it may narrow the passageway for urine flow, causing a variety of symptoms such as difficulty in starting the flow of urine, decreased force of the urinary stream, dribbling of urine, and increased frequency of urination. Occasionally, it may lead to a complete stopping of urine flow.

- Two drugs, Proscar (finasteride is the generic name) and Hytrin (terazosin), are being used to treat the symptoms of enlarged prostate glands. Clinical studies show the drugs offer significant symptom relief for enlarged prostate glands in about one of three men. Proscar does not seem to have any effect, either positive or negative, on prostate cancer.

- A new device called a Prostatron, which uses microwaves to kill excess prostate tisssue, has been approved by the Food and Drug Administration for treating BPH.

- Don't be alarmed by the statistics that say one in five men will get prostate cancer. That's your lifetime risk. If you are 40 years old, your chances of getting prostate cancer in the next 10 years is one in 1,000. Over the next 20 years, it's one in 100—but that's less than your risk of getting lung cancer.

- Early prostate cancer usually has no symptoms. Today, it is generally first detected by a PSA test—a blood test that detects prostate-specific antigen, a protein produced by the prostate gland.

- Early detection also includes a digital rectal examination that the doctor performs as part of a physical examination. Men should have a digital rectal exam each year after the age of 40.

- About 30 to 50 percent of men over 50 who have died from other causes were found to have cancerous cells in their prostates.

- Prostate cancer requires treatment depending on the stage of the disease, the age of the patient, and a full understanding of the treatments available.

• At the time prostate cancer is diagnosed, 50 to 65 percent of prostate cancers are localized, 9 to 17 percent have spread to the area near the prostate, and 20 to 25 percent have metastasized to other parts of the body.

• No treatment for prostate cancer is totally free of the possibility of some sexual or incontinence problems. It is important that treatment be discussed with and done under the guidance of a skilled, experienced doctor who specializes in that kind of treatment.

A VIEW INSIDE

What does the prostate look like?

The average adult prostate gland is about the size of a walnut. It also is designed somewhat like a walnut with sections bisected down the center by the urethra, which connects the bladder to the opening of the penis. Located below the bladder and in front of the rectum, it is divided into glandular zones—the peripheral, the central, and the transitional. The urethra, the tube that emerges from the bladder and carries urine, is surrounded by the prostate. The prostate gland is close to the front wall of the rectum, which is why it is possible for the physician to feel it with a finger during a rectal examination. Most prostate cancers are found in the peripheral zone.

> Just for the record: Prostate is often mispronounced as pros-trate, with the addition of an *r* in the last syllable. The correct pronunciation is "pros-tate," without the *r* in the second syllable.

What is the role of the prostate gland?

The prostate is a male sex gland, part of a man's reproductive system. Its major function is to provide the majority of the seminal fluid, which nourishes the sperm. The prostate needs male hormones to function. During ejaculation, the prostate gland squeezes fluid into the urethra to aid in the transport and nourishment of sperm.

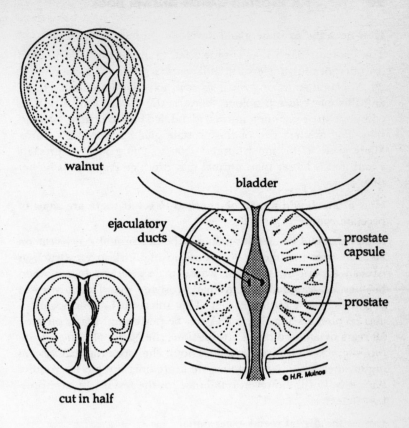

walnut

bladder

ejaculatory
ducts

prostate
capsule

prostate

© H.R. Mulnos

cut in half

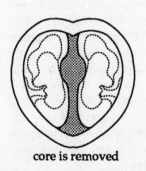

core is removed

**The prostate gland resembles
a walnut in its structure.**

How does the prostate gland develop?

The prostate gland weighs only a few grams at birth. At puberty it undergoes further growth and reaches adult size by about age 20. A second spurt of growth starts in most men at about age 40, and this may cause problems, because the growth will sometimes compress the remaining normal gland, leading to urinary obstruction. The average size of the prostate gland is about 30 grams. Many grow to be much larger—100 to 200 grams. A prostate gland that is larger than normal may produce PSA that is higher than average.

How often should a man be checked to see if there are signs of prostate cancer?

A digital rectal examination should be performed every year on all men over the age of 40. Those in high-risk groups, such as African Americans or those whose male relatives (e.g., father, brother, or grandfather) have had prostate cancer, are advised to begin the yearly testing earlier. The American Cancer Society is also recommending that a PSA test be performed yearly on men 50 years of age and older. At this time, the National Cancer Institute's screening information does not include routine PSA screening for men without symptoms. Medicare does not pay for routine PSA tests. It will, however, reimburse for the test if you have prostate cancer.

How is the digital rectal exam done?

Though not the most dignified of examinations, checking the prostate gland so that any abnormality can be detected early is an important part of any physical. The doctor may ask you to either bend from the hips with elbows on the examining table or to bend forward on your knees. Some doctors prefer to have the buttocks elevated in the knee–chest position. In either case, the doctor will ask you to bear down as the finger is inserted. It is normal to experience sensations of having to urinate or defecate during the examination. **However, if it hurts when the doctor touches your prostate, be sure to mention this. Pain can mean that you have prostatitis or inflammation of the prostate.**

What can the doctor tell about the prostate from the digital rectal exam?

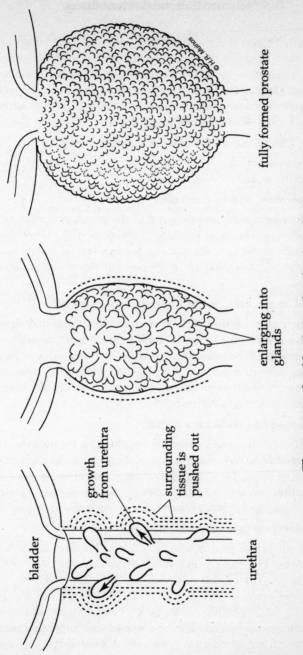

© H.R. Milnos

bladder

growth
from urethra

surrounding
tissue is
pushed out

urethra

enlarging into
glands

fully formed prostate

The prostate gland begins to develop in puberty and has another growth spurt in midlife.

The doctor is able to feel the prostate gland with a rubber-gloved finger inserted through the anus. To the experienced doctor, a cancerous lump feels hard, like a marble, in what is normally a fleshy gland. (Doctors say that a normal prostate feels like touching the tip of your nose and a suspicious lump feels like touching your elbow.) (See illustration on page 38.)

If I have a PSA exam, do I still need a digital exam?

Yes. Both exams together help your doctor to determine if there is a probability of cancer.

Are most prostate tumors cancerous?

No. The most common tumors found in the prostate are not cancerous. The most common prostate problem is BPH. More than three-quarters of men in the United States over 50 suffer from this enlargement, but only 10 to 20 percent develop significant obstruction.

Does blood in the urine mean I have prostate cancer?

Blood in the urine should never be ignored. Though it may signal prostate cancer, in most cases the blood comes from noncancerous enlargement of the prostate, infections in the bladder or prostate, broken blood vessels in the prostate, bladder tumors, or kidney stones. If there is blood in your urine, you should have a complete evaluation to determine the cause.

What does blood in the semen mean?

Blood in the semen should always be checked. In most cases, it is caused by an infection, inflammation of the prostate or surrounding seminal vesicles, or straining during a bowel movement or sexual or other activity. In some cases, it may be a warning sign of cancer. Your doctor can evaluate the cause easily and quickly.

Are there always symptoms with prostate cancer?

Some men who have prostate cancer report that they never had any symptoms. The same nonspecific symptoms that are caused by the enlargement of the prostate can also be caused by the growth of the prostate due to cancer. If the cancer has spread, there may be back, rib, hip, or shoulder pain; fatigue; weakness; or general aches and pains. The best way to find prostate cancer early is through regular digital exams and PSA testing.

POSSIBLE SYMPTOMS OF PROSTATE CANCER

Small prostate cancers often do not cause any symptoms. When symptoms do occur, they may include:

* Frequent urination, especially at night.
* Trouble starting or inability to hold back while urinating.
* A weak or interrupted urine flow.
* Pain or burning sensation during urination.
* Blood in the urine.
* Continuous pain in lower back, pelvis, or hips.

What is the difference between a benign and a malignant tumor?

A benign tumor is a growth that is not cancerous. It can usually be removed and in most cases does not come back. It does not spread to other parts of the body. Most benign tumors do not endanger your life unless they are growing in a confined area, such as the brain. On the other hand, malignant tumors are cancerous. The tumor cells do not organize themselves into normal patterns, and even though the tissue resembles the tissue of the normal cell, the arrangement of the cells is imperfect.

Why are cancerous cells so dangerous?

Cancerous cells deprive normal cells of nourishment and space. The cells build up into a mass of cells that compresses, invades, and destroys surrounding tissue.

Is it true that the more irregular the cells, the more malignant the tumor?

As a general rule, the more irregular or abnormal (doctors refer to it as undifferentiated) the cells look under the microscope, the more malignant the cancer. The greater the difference in appearance from a normal cell, the more active the cancer is likely to be and the more uncontrollable its course.

What is the difference between a differentiated and an undifferentiated cell?

Differentiated cells are cancerous cells that resemble normal cells. The more differentiated the cells, the less aggressive they are and

tumor grading

well differentiated → poorly differentiated

cells look abnormal and disorganized

cells resemble normal cells

prostate biopsies on microscope slides

© H.R. Mulnos

Difference between well-differentiated and poorly differentiated cancer cells.

the more likely the cancer is to respond to treatment. An undifferentiated cell, as you might expect, is more abnormal. The more undifferentiated (or abnormal) the cells appear under the microscope, the more cancerous the cells are and the more active and uncontrollable the cancer is likely to be. The aggressiveness of cells can vary from one area of the prostate to another. In prostate cancer, the cells are graded as: well, moderate, or poorly differentiated, and this factor is considered in determining the Gleason grade (see Chapter 5).

Can prostate cancer be inherited?

There is little known about the cause of prostate cancer, how to prevent it, or why it is nearly twice as common in black men as in white men. However, your risk rises steadily with the number of relatives you have with prostate cancer. If prostate cancer runs in your family, checkups should be started before age 40 and done regularly thereafter. There are a few studies that show fat in the diet may be associated with prostate cancer so family eating patterns may also play a role.

Are there any other studies being done on the subject of prostate cancer and diet or exercise?

Several studies have shown that eating an increased amount of fruits and vegetables may reduce a person's risk of getting cancer in general. A recent study suggests that three foods with a tomato base—tomato sauce, tomatoes, and pizza—all of which contain lycopene, may be especially beneficial regarding risk of prostate cancer. Another study indicated the importance of exercise— those men who had moderate or high exercise levels had lower rates of prostate cancer than those who did little or no exercise. However, these are early studies and more research needs to be done before any conclusions are reached.

Has a gene been identified for prostate cancer?

Two genes—KAI1 and E-cadherin—have been discovered that appear to be promising for prostate cancer. Although researchers are not clear at this time as to whether these genes will be able to predict the spread of prostate cancer or will be useful in the treatment of prostate cancer, they feel they may have some application with other prostate tumor markers in screening for prostate cancer. Many researchers are studying a variety of tumor markers that can help in both the original diagnosis of the disease as well as its spread. Using computer analysis, they are combining these biomarkers into tests that will in the future make it easier to determine the stage of the disease more easily and accurately.

How is the genetic makeup of a cancer cell determined?

The pathologist can measure the amount of DNA in a tumor cell by a technique called DNA flow cytometry. Normal cells have two copies of each chromosome. These cells are said to be diploid, which indicates that they have a normal amount of DNA per cell. If the cells are found to be aneuploid, this means there are abnormal amounts of DNA per cell. Men with diploid tumors appear to have a lower rate of spread or recurrence after treatment.

How many cells are in a cancerous tumor?

The number varies by the size of the tumor, the type of cell, and how fast the tumor is growing, sometimes called the doubling time. In many prostate cancers, the tumors grow very slowly. The tumor doubling time is slow, often taking months to years. Many men will not live long enough for the cancer to cause problems. Other men may have tumors that grow rapidly or that spread beyond the prostate. This variability is what sometimes makes it difficult to determine how to proceed and explains why it is so important to do proper testing in order to stage the cancer correctly .

What does it mean when the prostate cancer is encapsulated?

The true capsule of the prostate is the fibrous layer of tissue that surrounds the prostate. When the cancer is contained inside this area, the cancer is said to be encapsulated. If the cancer has pushed through this capsule, it may have spread to the nearest organs or it may involve the lymph nodes, the bones, or other parts of the body.

What does the doctor mean by the term margins?

The term margins refers to the area around the tumor. Clean margins means that in the area around the tumor no cancer cells are present—all cancer has been removed from the area.

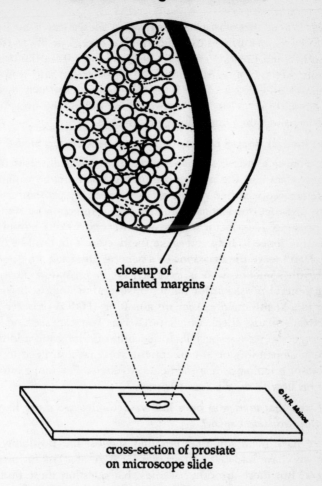

closeup of
painted margins

cross-section of prostate
on microscope slide

Cancer can penetrate the margins of the prostate.

What does it mean when I'm told my cancer is regionalized?

When the cancer is regionalized, it means that it has spread to
the region around the prostate but has not gone to other parts
of the body.

**What does it mean when the doctor says my cancer has metas-
tasized?**

When cancer metastasizes, it means that the cancer is no longer confined to one area of the body but has spread or has started to spread. When prostate cancer cells break away from the original tumor, they can spread through the bloodstream and lymphatic system to other parts of the body. The bones, especially those in the spine, hips, pelvis, and upper leg, as well as the liver, lungs, bladder, and other organs may be affected.

What kind of doctor is best for treating prostate problems?

A urologist, a doctor who specializes in treating diseases of the urinary tract and the male reproductive system, is best qualified to determine whether symptoms are caused by prostate cancer, BPH, or some other condition, such as an infection or stones in the prostate. This doctor will have the necessary skills, equipment, and experience to help you make the decisions that will be facing you. **Don't leave the decisions to a general physician.** You need to deal with someone who is experienced in prostate cancer. Ask your general physician for names of several urologists. If you belong to a health maintenance organization (HMO) or other managed care plans, check which physicians you can see and what coverage you have, especially for second opinions and additional testing. Depending on the treatment, you may also need to see a radiation oncologist or a medical oncologist. For more information on how to do this, see Chapter 7.

Is it true that men who have had vasectomies are more likely to develop prostate cancer?

There have been some studies that suggest the possibility that men who have had vasectomies may be at greater risk for prostate cancer. But there are other studies that question these findings. An expert committee convened by the National Institutes of Health has found that the association, at most, is a small one. Further studies are needed to determine whether or not vasectomy is associated with prostate cancer in any way.

NONCANCEROUS CONDITIONS

What causes infection and inflammation of the prostate gland and prostatic urethra?

Infection and inflammation can be caused by bacterial or non-bacterial infections or because of inadequate emptying of fluids normally manufactured in the prostate gland. Most often, the infection is caused by the viruslike organism clamydia, but it may be caused by other organisms transmitted through oral, vaginal, or anal intercourse. Infection is caused by bacteria or some other microorganism. Inflammation will often occur without infection.

What are the symptoms of infection or inflammation of the prostate gland and the prostatic urethra?

The most common symptoms are:

- A small brown or yellow stain on underclothing.
- A watery discharge at the opening of the penis in the morning upon arising.
- An itchy sensation inside the penis.
- Discomfort within the penis after urinating.
- A deeper feeling of discomfort, which may indicate that the infection is affecting the prostatic urethra (within the prostate gland).
- There may also be pain in the perineum (the area between the scrotum and the anus), in the rectum, or in the area just above the pubic hairline.

What treatments are used for infections and inflammation of the prostate gland?

Treatment will depend upon the exact diagnosis: whether the doctor finds that you have nonspecific urethritis, chronic bacterial prostatitis, or nonbacterial prostatitis (prostatosis). The first two will usually be treated with drugs—often antibiotics—and the third can be treated by encouraging you to empty the prostate gland through intercourse or masturbation.

What is nonbacterial prostatitis?

Nonbacterial prostatitis is caused by an accumulation of prostatic fluid in the prostate gland caused by a sudden decrease in the frequency of ejaculation. It can usually be relieved by increased sexual intercourse or masturbation. It can be directly related to a change in sexual habits.

What is acute bacterial prostatitis?

This very uncommon condition results from a sudden rush of bacteria into the prostate gland either from an infection in the urethra or from an infection somewhere else in the body. Usually it is accompanied by a fever, flulike aches and pains, and low-abdominal or low-back pain. Swelling of the prostate causes the inside diameter of the prostatic urethra to narrow, making urination difficult or impossible, and may require a temporary catheter. Sometimes appendicitis or the passage of a kidney stone down the ureter and toward the bladder may be the cause of similar symptoms.

What does pain in the pelvis or penis mean?

Often this condition, referred to by doctors as prostatodynia, has many of the symptoms of prostatitis, but no evidence of infection or inflammation can be found. The cause is usually tension in the muscles that surround the prostate and rectum. It is sometimes seen in cyclists who spend many hours on a narrow racing seat or in men who have tension headaches. Treatment with alpha blockers, balloon dilation, muscle relaxants, and hot baths may be prescribed.

What is BPH?

In simple terms, this condition means that you have an enlarged prostate. About three-quarters of men over 50 and 80 percent of men over 80 have enlarged prostates.

Why does BPH cause prostate problems?

When a man is in his forties, the prostate gland begins to enlarge. The new growth (or hyperplasia) may occur part or most of the way around the prostatic urethra. It does not always grow symmetrically. There may be more new growth on one side than on the other or on the bottom rather than on the sides. Furthermore, the new growth will usually have more fibrous and muscular tissue. If it grows outward, it tends to compress the capsule of the prostate. Often it grows inward as well, causing the narrowing of the channel through which the urine flows. The prostate enlarged by BPH can cause the normal levels of PSA to double.

What is TURP?

TURP is the abbreviation for transurethral resection of the prostate. This operation involves the endoscopic removal of tissue to relieve blockage due to BPH. It is done through the penis. It is major surgery that may result in complications such as retrograde ejaculation, impotence, or incontinence. It is not considered to be a procedure that should be used for the diagnosis of cancer, which should be made by needle biopsy if feasible. If you have prostate cancer and need treatment for severe obstructive urinary symptoms, you should be advised to have treatment that deals with the cancerous problem. Sometimes you may need a TURP as part of your cancer treatment because of obstruction. This operation costs $8,000 to $12,000. You are usually in the hospital for about three days.

What if my prostate cancer was found during a TURP for BPH?

In some cases, after TURP surgery, the biopsy will disclose signs of cancer. Because it may take up to three months for the site to heal completely, it is important that if either a radical prostatectomy or radiation is decided upon as treatment for the prostate cancer, it be postponed for six to eight weeks to minimize complications.

What is TUIP?

TUIP stands for transurethral incision of the prostate. This operation involves incisions in the bladder neck to relieve blockage of obstructions due to BPH. The biggest advantage to this procedure over a TURP is that it has fewer complications and leads to retrograde ejaculation much less frequently than TURP.

What is retrograde ejaculation?

Retrograde ejaculation is when the semen flows back into the bladder instead of coming out the end of the penis. This causes the semen to mix with the urine in the bladder. In certain circumstances, the semen may be recovered for artificial insemination by catheterizing after ejaculation and recovering the semen from the bladder.

If I have undergone surgery for a benign tumor of the prostate, does this mean I can no longer have prostate cancer?

No. Most operations performed for prostate problems other than cancer do not remove the entire prostate. Unless you have undergone a total prostatectomy, you should understand that it is still possible to develop prostate cancer. Remaining prostatic tissue must be examined by your physician as part of your annual medical examination.

Are drugs used to treat symptoms of enlarged prostate glands?

Two drugs, Proscar (finasteride) and Hytrin (terazosin), are being used to treat symptoms of enlarged prostate glands. Proscar shrinks the prostate. Hytrin relaxes muscle tissue and helps lessen the blockage. Proscar also reduces PSA, so you need to have a PSA test before you begin to use it and about six months later. If your PSA level has not dropped by a third or a half after taking the Proscar for several months, you may have prostate cancer or another problem. Hytrin does not change your PSA value. The drugs cost hundreds of dollars a year.

Are microwaves ever used in treating BPH?

Yes, there is a new device, called a Prostatron, that uses microwaves to heat the enlarged prostate to kill excess prostate tissue. A catheter is threaded through the urethra, and using computers, microwaves heat the prostate. You do not feel any heat because cooling water is circulated inside the catheter. No anesthesia is needed, and the treatment takes about an hour to complete. There are few side effects, although about one in three men has swelling that does not allow urination for up to three days, but catheters can be used during this period. The device treats the symptoms of BPH, such as urgency, frequency, straining, and intermittent flow, but it does not correct the problems of not being able to completely empty your bladder or of having a weak urinary stream. Because of the design of the Prostatron, it can be used only on men with medium-sized prostates. Surgery is still the most effective treatment but you must undergo anesthesia, and you may have blood loss, impotence, and other complications. Surgery also costs about twice as much as the new microwave treatment, which gives you another alternative if you cannot or do not wish to have an operation. Studies are continuing to look at long-term side effects and the need for retreatment.

chapter 4

What Other Tests Will I Need?

After discovering you have an elevated PSA, the next question that needs to be answered is, "Do I need more tests?" Many factors are involved. Depending on the numbers, some doctors take a wait-and-see stance. Others feel it is important to proceed to a biopsy to find out if cancer is present. Other testing may be needed to make a definitive diagnosis. Doctors can detect small irregularities and biopsy them accurately using ultrasound. Depending on your PSA level, a bone scan, magnetic resonance imaging (MRI), or a computerized tomography (CT) scan may be done.

What are the guidelines for proceeding with more tests?

Different doctors will make these decisions in different ways. Here are possible guidelines for how to proceed, suggested by our discussions with a number of physicians:

- **If the digital rectal exam is normal and the PSA is less than 4 (6.5 for men over 70):** No treatment. Schedule an annual or semiannual recheck.

- If the digital exam is abnormal and the PSA is under 4 (6.5 for men over 70): An ultrasound exam with biopsies of the abnormal area.
- If the digital exam is normal, but the PSA is over 4 (6.5 for men over 70): The choice is usually either a decision to repeat the PSA in three months or an immediate ultrasound with biopsies. (A steadily rising PSA is more indicative of cancer than is a one-time high reading.)
- If the PSA is over 10: Schedule an ultrasound with biopsies.

QUESTIONS TO ASK IF THE DOCTOR SUSPECTS PROSTATE CANCER

- Were the PSA test results elevated?
- What was the PSA reading?
- How high was my PSA level above normal?
- If this was your first PSA test, ask, Could I wait three months and have another PSA test before making any decisions?
- What sort of lump did you feel?
- Is the prostate enlarged or is there a definite nodule or ridge?
- Where was it located?
- Will the biopsy be done with an ultrasound probe?
- Will I need an operation to check my lymph nodes?

What do I need to know when the doctor suggests further testing?

In most cases, the doctor will want to do further testing to determine why your reading is high. First will be a thorough digital exam to see if there are any abnormal hard or raised areas on your prostate. To help figure out the meaning of the elevated PSA, the doctor will usually suggest that a biopsy and other tests be done.

BIOPSIES

What is a biopsy?

A biopsy is the procedure in which a piece of tissue is obtained and examined under the microscope to determine whether can-

---

MOST COMMON TESTS THAT MAY BE USED TO HELP DIAGNOSE YOUR PROSTATE CANCER

- Digital rectal exam.
- PSA level.
- Prostatic acid phosphatase (PAP) test.
- Ultrasound screening.
- Biopsy.
- Urinalysis.
- Cystoscopy.
- Bone scan.
- CT scan.
- Lymph node analysis.
- MRI.

---

cer is present. For the prostate, several minute pieces of tissues are taken. The biopsy is read by a pathologist, a physician who specializes in the study of normal and diseased body tissues. When looked at under the microscope, normal cells have an orderly appearance. The cells from each organ carry a different genetic message that determines their structure and function. Cancer cells have an appearance that is more disorganized than normal cells.

Are there different kinds of biopsies taken for prostate cancer?

There are several kinds. A transrectal biopsy (the needle is inserted through the wall of the rectum) is the most common one used today. Transperineal biopsies (the needle is inserted under the scrotum) are sometimes used in men who may be at high risk for complications with a transrectal biopsy. Both can be done with an ultrasound and a biopsy gun with a fine needle. Aspirational biopsies (the tissue is taken through a syringe) and core biopsies (with a heavier needle) are not usually used.

How is a biopsy for prostate cancer done?

In the past, a finger-guided needle biopsy was used or a surgical procedure was required. Today, most doctors with up-to-date

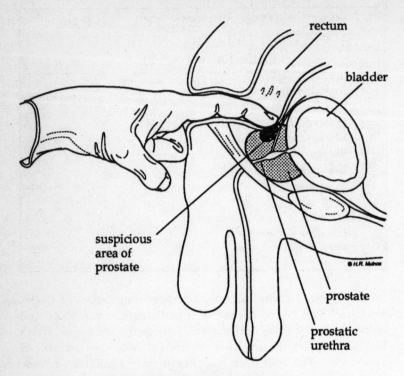

rectum

bladder

suspicious
area of
prostate

© H.R. Mulnos

prostate

prostatic
urethra

**The examining finger in the rectum
can feel a hard or suspicious area.
The examining finger cannot feel
the middle lobe of the prostate.**

equipment will obtain needle biopsies using ultrasound probes,
which ensure a more accurate method of obtaining biopsy readings. **Before having a biopsy, check with the doctor to be sure
your biopsy will be done with ultrasound probes. Also, if this is
your first PSA test, inquire if it would be advisable to wait three
months and do a second PSA test before having a biopsy.**

Why is ultrasound the best way to diagnose prostate cancer?

Most urologists feel that using ultrasound is a superior way of
diagnosing very early prostate cancer because it can detect smaller
cancers more accurately. It also enables the urologist to get sam-

ples from selected areas of the prostate. The ultrasound probe is often able to discover cancerous tissue that is missed by a digital examination. In addition, the extent of any possible spread beyond the prostate gland can sometimes be visualized on the ultrasound screen. If there is no cancer and the problem is BPH, the size of the prostate gland can be seen, making it possible for the physician to make surgical decisions based on the size of the prostate.

What kind of doctor usually does the ultrasound exam?

Ultrasound may be done by a diagnostic radiologist in a hospital, but most urologists are now including this as part of their office procedures.

How is an ultrasound-guided needle biopsy done?

In preparation for the biopsy procedure, you will be asked to have an enema to help remove fecal material so the ultrasound will be clear. A lubricated probe will be placed in the rectum. The probe bounces high-frequency sound waves into the prostate. The different densities between normal prostate tissue and cancer show up as shadows on the ultrasound image. The surgeon guides a spring-loaded device that fires a thin, long needle through the wall of the rectum into the prostate. The needle, which can be seen on the screen as it is moved into each area, opens inside the prostate, captures a bit of the prostate tissue, and closes. The needle is then withdrawn so the sample can be removed and analyzed.

How many biopsies are usually taken?

There is some controversy among physicians about how many biopsy ''punches'' should be taken. Most doctors take six to eight random biopsies from different areas if there is no area that appears to be highlighted. Other doctors feel that additional biopsies should be taken in deeper areas of the prostate. If a problem area is seen, additional biopsies will be taken.

Does it hurt to have an ultrasound-directed biopsy?

You may feel a bit uncomfortable for a few seconds when the doctor puts the probe in, especially if you have had surgery for hemorrhoids. The device that fires the needle is so rapid that it is virtually painless. Some 5 to 10 percent of patients feel a little ache when the gun is fired. Anesthesia is not used, although some doctors will use anesthetic jelly when inserting the probe. You can usually return home when the procedure is completed. Most doctors will advise you to have someone drive you because you may be somewhat sore and uncomfortable.

What do I need to do to prepare for an ultrasound biopsy?

Usually your doctor will advise you to stop taking aspirin or any pills that contain aspirin a week or more before having a biopsy. In addition, you should be off any anti-inflammatory pills (such as Advil and Motrin) a few days before the biopsy. If you are taking a blood thinner (such as Coumadin), you need to talk with your doctor about how you should proceed with the biopsy. It would be wise to tell your doctor about any medication you are taking before the biopsy is scheduled.

Are there any aftereffects of an ultrasound biopsy?

You can continue your normal activities the day after your biopsy, although some doctors will advise you not to drink alcohol for a few days. You may see some blood in your urine or your bowel movements. Bleeding will usually stop after a week or two. You may also see blood in your ejaculate for a few months as a result of the biopsy.

Is the ultrasound exam safe?

Yes. Ultrasound uses sound waves to produce the picture. No radiation is used in an ultrasound exam.

How much does an ultrasound biopsy of the prostate cost?

The cost depends upon what part of the country you live in, where the biopsy is done, and how many health professsionals are involved in the test. The cost can range from a few hundred dollars to over a thousand.

Does the pathologist who examines the tissue need special training?

In order to be certified by the American Board of Pathology, the person must be a licensed doctor of medicine or osteopathy and have several years of specialized training and experience. In these days of changing technology and with new instrumentation and new testing mechanisms, it is essential that the pathologist be well trained and an expert in the cancer field. As in other specialties, the skill and competence of pathologists vary. A decision regarding whether cancer is the disease in the tissue being examined depends on the interpretation one individual pathologist makes of the cellular structure of the biopsy.

Should I have another opinion on the biopsy?

Often the specimens are sent to experts in larger institutions for consultation, especially if the pathologist is practicing alone in a small community. If your diagnosis is based on the single pathological report of a single pathologist in a small community, be sure to ask that a consultation with other pathologists be arranged. (This may be a little difficult in these days of managed care, but you need to discuss the possibilities with your doctor.) Also important is the relationship between your doctor and the pathologist. They need to be talking with each other and working together as a team.

When can I expect to get the results of my biopsy?

It depends on the laboratory, the time of the week you are having the test done, and the lab's work schedule. The results usually come back to your doctor within two to four days. Make sure you ask your doctor when and how you will be given the results.

Can I have an ultrasound without having a biopsy?

No. About 20 percent of the time, although cancer is present, it is not detected on the ultrasound. If you have an elevated PSA or the doctor has felt something on your prostate, a biopsy will be done even if the ultrasound does not find anything. On the other hand, you normally would not have been scheduled for an ultrasound if the doctor had not felt an abnormality in doing the digital exam or if your PSA was not elevated.

What if the biopsy shows I do not have cancer, but my PSA still is high?

As with other tests, biopsies are not 100 percent accurate. About 15 percent of them show no cancer when cancer is indeed present. It may be that the cancer cells are in a part of the prostate that was not tested by the biopsy. Or you may have a problem that is not cancer that is causing your PSA to rise. In any case, you will need some follow-up. Your doctor will order some other exams and may need to repeat your PSA test in a few months to see if the level has changed. Another biopsy may need to be done.

Won't the biopsy cause the cancer to spread?

There is no evidence that a biopsy causes cancer to spread.

OTHER TESTS

What other techniques are used to determine if there is cancer?

An intravenous pyelogram (IVP), which is a series of x-rays of the organs of the urinary tract, may be ordered. The doctor may also order urine tests and may look into the urethra and bladder through a thin lighted tube called a cystoscope. Depending upon the initial findings, further testing, such as an excretory urogram, renal scan, and bone scan, using CT or MRI, may be necessary.

How is an IVP done?

An IVP (also referred to as an excretory urogram) is an x-ray study of the urinary tract. An iodine-containing substance is injected into a vein in your arm. It concentrates in the kidney and causes the urinary tract to become opaque, outlining the urine-filled ducts of the kidney, ureters, and bladder. A series of x-rays is taken during the approximately 30-minute period when the substance is in the body. This test may be done to determine if there is any involvement of the cancer in some of the adjoining structures. It is helpful to determine how well the bladder is emptied during voiding, to see if there is any obstruction to the drainage of the kidneys caused by the enlarged prostate gland, and to see how large the prostate gland is by observing the shadow it casts within the bladder. (Note: The substance injected for the IVP may cause a reaction in those with known allergies to iodine and iodine products.)

What does the doctor learn from urine tests?

Urine tests provide the doctor with a great deal of information about the genitourinary tract even though alone they cannot provide a definite diagnosis. If the urinalysis contains white blood cells (more than one to three per high-power microscopic field), it can indicate an infection. The presence of red blood cells (anything over zero to two per high-power field) can signal anything from a mild inflammation in the urethra or bladder to the possibility of cancer.

What's the right way for me to prepare for a urine specimen?

The most accurate urine culture is from the middle portion of the urinary stream. You will be asked to void the first few ounces of urine into the toilet, collect the middle portion of the stream into a sterile container, and finish directly into the toilet. Do not stop or interrupt the urinary stream in the process. (Uncircumcised men should retract the foreskin and clean the penis well with soap and water before starting to urinate for a urine specimen.)

How is a cystoscopy done?

A cystoscopy is done with a hollow instrument that is inserted in the penile urethra and then into the bladder. The pencil-thin, lighted instrument allows the doctor to view the urethra, bladder, prostate, and kidneys. You will lie on your back with your knees bent, legs apart, and feet or thighs supported as the doctor inserts the instrument, usually using local anesthetic jelly. A sterile solution is put through the scope to expand the bladder and give the doctor a clear view. You may feel fullness or the need to urinate. A catheter is sometimes left in place to drain urine until swelling in the urethra subsides. Most men report that the description of the procedure is much worse than the actual test.

Are there any aftereffects to having a cystoscopy?

You may need to urinate often, and you may have a burning sensation during and after urination. Drink lots of liquids to prevent infection. You also may have pinkish urine for a few days. If your urine is red with blood clots, if you do not urinate within eight hours after the test, or if you have a high fever, chills, or pain, you should report these symptoms to your doctor.

What is a bone scan?

A bone scan is a nuclear scan that uses a radioactive substance to diagnose whether your prostate cancer has spread to your bones.

OTHER TESTS THAT MAY BE USED IN DIAGNOSING PROSTATE CANCER

TEST	PROCEDURE
Intravenous pyelogram (IVP)	You may need to fast and take laxatives before test. You will lie on your back on x-ray table for preliminary film, then contrast material will be injected in a vein in your arm. You will need to be still while x-rays are taken, usually at 5-minute intervals.
Cystoscopy	A lighted instrument is inserted into the urethra and bladder. If being done under local anesthetic, drink plenty of fluids; otherwise no food or drink for 8 hours before the test. The test takes about 15–45 minutes. If it done as an outpatient procedure, it is uncomfortable and you should plan to have someone drive you home.
Bone scan	Radioactive material is injected into an arm vein and travels through the bloodstream to the bone. You will need to drink several glasses of fluid before the scan. You will lie on your back or change positions as a large camera scans back and forth above you. The procedure itself takes about 1 hour, but you must wait 2 to 3 hours after the material is injected before the scan can be done.
Computerized tomography (CT scan)	You may be asked to fast for 4 hours before the test. Contrast dye is either swallowed, injected into your arm or given through an enema. You will lie on a table with the part of your body to be tested positioned in the middle of a large ring. The table moves every few seconds as the machine takes a new slice of pictures. The large scanning machine moves around you. You need to lie very still and hold your breath while the images are being taken. It takes about an hour. *(continued)*

OTHER TESTS THAT MAY BE USED IN DIAGNOSING PROSTATE CANCER *(cont)*	
TEST	**PROCEDURE**
Magnetic resonance imaging (MRI)	An MRI is similar to a CT scan but uses magnetics instead of x-rays. The contrast material may be given through a vein. The scan takes from 30 minutes to 2 hours. If you have claustrophobia, discuss it with the radiologist beforehand, since the equipment may enclose you from head to thighs with the wall of the chamber only a few inches from your face. If you have an aneurysm, pacemaker, implanted pump, or other metallic implant, you should discuss this with your doctor since the magnetic pull of the MRI is very strong and can cause problems.
Renal scan	Material is injected into an arm vein, and travels through the bloodstream to the kidneys. You sit up or lie on your back while a large camera scans as the material circulates through the kidneys. The test takes about 1 hour. You may need to return in 4 hours or later for additional scans. More than one radioactive material may be injected. You will need to empty your bladder after the test.

A small amount of radioactive material, injected into your arm vein, travels through the bloodstream to your bones. A special camera scans your body, creating an image of your skeleton.

How long does it take to do a bone scan?

The scan itself takes about an hour. However, you will have to wait about two to three hours after the radioactive material is injected to give it a chance to spread to your bones. You will need to drink four to six glasses of water during that time to flush out of your body any material not being picked up by the bones.

Before the scan is done, you will be asked to empty your bladder. You will lie on your back or change positions as the large camera scans back and forth above you.

Will I need to go to a hospital to get a bone scan?

Yes. The nuclear machinery is a major investment so that most bone scans are done in hospitals. The scans are usually done by a technician and interpreted by a nuclear medicine physician, in the hospital radiology or nuclear medicine department.

When will I be able to resume my normal activities?

In most cases you will be able to go back to your usual activities and diet immediately after your bone scan. You will not need to stay overnight in the hospital. It will usually take a few days before the doctor who ordered the scan will know the results. Ask the doctor who sends you for the test when you can call for results.

How much does a bone scan cost?

As with other tests, the cost of a bone scan depends on where you live and where the scan is done. It ranges from $500 to over $1,000.

What is a CT scan?

CT stands for computerized tomography. A scanner passes a pencil-thin beam of x-rays through a selected part of your body, creating a 360° picture of that slice in a few seconds. The information is processed in a computer, which shows the image on a TV screen. The pictures are much more detailed than regular x-rays. CT scans are usually done if you are going to have radiation treatment for your prostate cancer. They are not usually done if you are going to have a radical prostatectomy. The cost of a CT scan ranges from $600 to $1,500, depending upon where you live and where the scan is done.

How is the CT scan done?

The test is usually done in the diagnostic radiology department of a hospital or a medical office. It is performed by an x-ray technician and interpreted by a qualified diagnostic radiologist. You will lie on a table with the part of your body to be tested positioned in the middle of a large ring. You will be alone in the room, but you will be able to talk to the technician who will be watching through a window in the room. You will be asked to lie very still and hold your breath while the pictures are being taken. The table will move a little bit every few seconds as the machine takes a new slice of pictures. A large scanning machine moves around you. You may hear a buzzing or a clicking sound. When the test is finished, you should be able to go back to your normal routine and diet.

What is an MRI?

An MRI is a scanner with a large cylinder that records water molecules in the body using magetic properties of protons in hydrogen atoms to create cross-sectional images of the body. An MRI creates sectional images of the body, similar to CT scans, but it does not expose you to any radiation. Men who have an aneurysm, pacemaker, implanted pump, or other metallic implant should be sure to let their doctors know of these problems if an MRI is suggested. The cost of an MRI is about $750 to $1,500.

How is the MRI done?

An MRI is usually done in a special room, part of the hospital's nuclear medicine or diagnostic radiology department. You will be asked to remove any metal objects that might be attracted to the magnet. You may be given a contrast dye through a vein. You will lie on a table, secured by straps. The table will move into the opening of the narrow cylindrical chamber with the lower part of your body positioned in the center of the magnet. Some people find the process very confining. It may also be noisy. You may find it helpful to bring your earphones and listen to music during the procedure. If you have claustophobia, you should discuss the problem with your doctor, who may suggest that you take a sedative before the test. The procedure takes anywhere from 30 minutes to two or more hours.

What is endorectal coil MRI?

This is a new test that checks if the cancer has spread locally beyond the confines of the prostate. A special coil is placed in the rectum that gives more detailed images when MRI is used. Researchers feel that this new test could help to identify the men who are at high risk for prostate cancer that spreads into the areas beyond the site of the tumor.

What is a renal scan?

A renal scan is another method of visualizing the urinary tract. It is used less often than the excretory urogram in detecting prostate cancer but is an excellent technique for evaluating whether there is any obstruction of the drainage of the kidneys. A radioactive material is injected intravenously and a gamma camera is used to pick up signals from the tracer material to create an image.

What does the doctor learn from the various types of tests that are done?

The tests are done to give your doctor a picture of what is happening in the prostate and whether there is any sign that the cancer has spread to other areas. The biopsy is especially important because it can help to grade the cancer and provide guidelines for treatment.

What is laparoscopic lymph node dissection?

This is a technique that makes it possible for the physician to remove and examine the pelvic lymph nodes without a major operation. Four small incisions are made in the lower abdominal wall so that lymph nodes can be removed. A small TV camera makes it possible for the surgeon to remove the nodes and examine them for cancerous cells. As part of the testing process, lymph node dissection is another tool that may help reveal information about whether the cancer has spread, although some doctors feel that it may give only minimal information except in the most expert of hands. There is more information about lymph node dissection in Chapter 8.

chapter 5

Understanding the Diagnosis

Once all the testing is completed, you will have a better understanding of the status of your prostate and how serious the threat of cancer is. Prostate cancer, unlike many other cancers, does not, in most cases, progress in a rapid fashion. This gives you time to make a thoughtful decision about what to do next. You need to know clearly exactly what the diagnosis is.

QUESTIONS TO ASK ABOUT YOUR DIAGNOSIS

- What is my PSA level?
- What is the PSA density?
- What is my Gleason grade?
- What is the DNA status?
- What is my type of cancer?
- What is the stage of my disease?
- What size is my prostate gland?
- Where in the prostate is the cancer located?
- What are my possible treatment options?

What is the Gleason grade?

The Gleason grade is a method used by doctors to determine how close to normal the cells look when the tissue is examined under the microscope. Though the following may be hard for the lay-person to translate, the system recognizes the following five patterns of cells:

1. Closely packed, single, separate, round, uniform glands; well-defined tumor margin.

2. Single, separate, round, less uniform glands separated by stroma up to one gland in diameter; tumor margin less well defined.

3. Single, separate, irregular glands of variable size; enlarged masses with cribriform or papillary pattern; poorly defined tumor margin.

4. Fused glands in mass with infiltrating cords, small glands with papillary, cribriform, or solid patterns; small, dark, or hyper-nephroid cells (clear cells).

5. Few or no glands in background of masses with comedo pattern; cords or sheets of tumor cells infiltrating stroma.

How is the Gleason grade determined?

The grade is determined by assigning one number to the most prominent pattern of your cells and another to the secondary pattern and adding the two together. The total can be anywhere from 2 (1 + 1) to 10 (5 + 5).

What do the Gleason grades mean?

The grades measure differentiation, the medical term used to describe how closely cancer cells resemble their normal counterparts. Grades 2 to 4 indicate that the tumor is well differentiated, 5 to 7 indicate that it is moderately differentiated, and 8 to 10 indicate that it is poorly differentiated.

What is meant by well differentiated?

Cancer cells are described as well differentiated when they look much like normal cells of the same type and are able to carry out some functions of normal cells. Poorly differentiated and undifferentiated tumor cells are disorganized and abnormal looking.

GLEASON GRADES	
Gleason 2, 3, 4	Most like normal cells, well differentiated, slow growing, low probability of metastasis, low grade
Gleason 5, 6, 7	Can behave like normal cells or like aggressive cells, moderately differentiated, moderate probability of metastasis, moderate grade
Gleason 8, 9, 10	Least like normal cells, poorly differentiated, high probability of metastasis, high grade

As a general rule, the more the cells look like normal cells under the microscope, the slower growing they are. The greater the difference in the appearance of the cell from what is normal, the higher the number that is assigned on the Gleason grade.

What does the Gleason grade mean in terms of deciding on treatment?

The Gleason grading can be valuable in helping to make decisions about the type of treatment chosen. It is another measurement when added to the PSA and digital exam that can help in coming to a conclusion about treatment.

Are there other grading systems?

There have been some 30 grading systems proposed, but most have not been universally accepted. You may hear of a system based on the slight variations in the size of the nuclear structure of the cell that uses only three grades:

> **Grade 1** = Low grade, slightly enlarged nuclei.
> **Grade 2** = Medium grade.
> **Grade 3** = High grade, loss of cell cohesion, large variation in size of nuclei.

Is the grade of cancer similar to the stage of cancer?

No. They are two different measurements. Grade is a single measurement used to describe how closely cancer cells resemble their normal counterparts. Stage (see Stage and Treatment Choices for Prostate Cancer) takes into account the various components of what is known about your cancer and how far it has progressed so that the doctor can determine what treatment is most appropriate.

What features help to determine whether my prostate cancer is a more or less serious disease?

There are a number of different criteria that help to determine which prostate cancers are likely to be more serious. They include the volume or size, the Gleason grade, the pattern of growth, the serum PSA, and the area where the cancer is located. All of these criteria are important to take into account when making decisions about what treatment will be used.

What type of cancer are most prostate cancers?

Over 95 percent of prostate cancers that are confined to the prostate gland are adenocarcinomas that vary in appearance and differentiation. The remainder are usually squamous cell or sarcomas. Most of these are found in the posterior lobe and are usually multifocal.

Does location of the cancer in the prostate make a difference?

The prostate is divided into three zones. Next to the urethra is the transitional zone. This is surrounded by a large shell of glandular tissue called the peripheral zone, where most cancers start. Surrounding the ejaculatory ducts is the central zone. Cancers in the peripheral, or outer, area are considered more serious. Cancers in the transitional, or inner, area are at lowest risk. If the cancer has penetrated the capsule and has gone into surrounding connective tissue, it will be categorized in a higher stage than one that is contained inside the capsule.

Does my age make a difference in determining what treatment will be used?

Yes, it does. Younger men who have no other serious illnesses are more likely to die from their prostate cancers. On the other hand, older men, especially those with localized tumors, are more likely

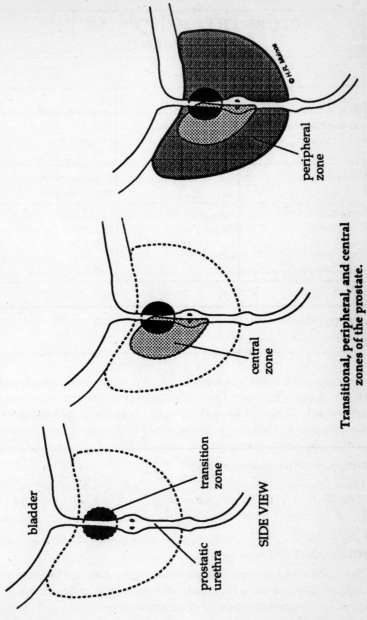

bladder

transition zone

prostatic urethra

SIDE VIEW

central zone

peripheral zone

Transitional, peripheral, and central zones of the prostate.

FACTORS THAT HELP DETERMINE TREATMENT

FACTOR	LESS SERIOUS	MORE SERIOUS
Tumor size or volume	Small	Large
Grade/Gleason score	Well differentiated 2–4	Moderate or poorly differentiated 5–10
Growth pattern	Confined to prostate	Extracapsular or with positive margins
PSA level Age 40–49 Age 50–59 Age 60–69 Age 70–79	**Normal** Under 2.5 Under 3.5 Under 4.5 Under 6.5	**Elevated** Over 2.5 Over 3.5 Over 4.5 Over 6.5
Tumor stage	I–II	III–IV
Location of tumor	Inner area (transitional)	Outer area (peripheral)

never to suffer any real disabilities from their prostate cancer and to die of other illnesses. Doctors usually treat younger men more aggressively, although some doctors are using watchful waiting for sexually active younger men diagnosed with early-stage prostate cancer with low Gleason scores.

How is prostate cancer staged?

There are several classifications used to stage prostate cancer, including the TNM system, and systems that use the letters A to D or the numbers I to IV. The one most commonly used is the Stage I to IV system.

What is the TNM system?

The TNM method is an international system that can be used to compare the results of treatment worldwide. It uses Stages I to IV based on the assessment of three components:

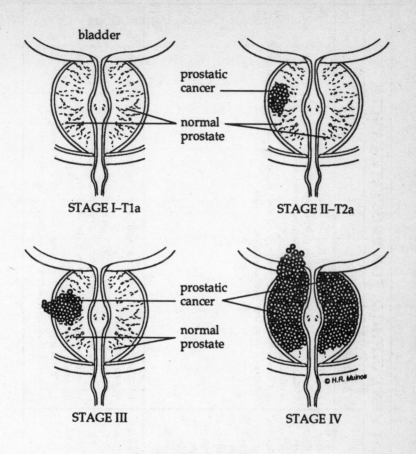

bladder

prostatic cancer

normal prostate

STAGE I–T1a

STAGE II–T2a

prostatic cancer

normal prostate

STAGE III

STAGE IV

© H.R. Muinos

Different stages of prostate cancer.

Stage I–T1a:
Cancer cannot be felt or seen by imaging.
Found through PSA, ultrasound, or
accidentally during surgery.

Stage I–T2a:
Cancer found only in prostate gland.

Stage III:
Cancer cells have spread outside the covering
(capsule) of prostate to tissues surrounding it.

Stage IV:
Cancer cells have spread to lymph nodes or to
organs and tissues outside prostate.

STAGE AND TREATMENT CHOICES FOR PROSTATE CANCER

STAGE	DESCRIPTION	TREATMENT
STAGE I T1a, T1b, or T1c, N0, M0 Stage A1, A2	Cancer is confined to the prostate. It cannot be felt and there are no symptoms. It's found through PSA, ultrasound, or accidentally when surgery is done for other reasons. T1a involves one area of the prostate and is well differentiated. In T1b, cancer cells are moderately or poorly differentiated or involve multiple foci in the gland. In T1c, the cancer has been identified by needle biopsy because of an elevated PSA.	1. Careful observation without further immediate treatment. 2. External radiation (should be delayed 4–6 weeks if a TURP was performed). 3. Radical prostatectomy with or without nerve-sparing technique usually with lymphadenectomy. 4. Clinical trials: radiation seeding, external radiation using three-dimensional conformal treatment planning or other trials.
Stage II T2a, T2b, T2c, N0, M0 Stage B1, B2	Cancer can be felt during a rectal exam. Cancer cells are found only in the prostate gland. T2a involves half a lobe or less. T2b involves more than half a lobe but not both lobes. T2c involves both lobes of the gland.	1. Radical prostatectomy with or without nerve-sparing technique, usually with lymphadenectomy. 2. External radiation (delayed 4–6 weeks if a TURP was performed). 3. Careful observation without further immediate treatment in selected cases. When disease progresses, hormonal therapy may be used, followed by radiation treatment if needed. 4. Clinical trials: radiation seeding, external radiation using three-dimensional conformal treatment planning, cryosurgery, or other trials.

Stage III T3, N0, M0 Stage C	Cancer cells have spread outside the covering (capsule) of the prostate to the tissues surrounding it. Seminal vesicles may have cancer in them. T3c is cancer that has spread to the seminal vesicles.	Symptoms, age, and other illnesses need to be considered in making treatment decisions. 1. External radiation with linear accelerator (delayed 4–6 weeks if a TURP was performed). 2. Radical prostatectomy with lymphadenectomy followed by radiation if capsular penetration or seminal vesicle invasion found during operation or if level of PSA is detectable 3 weeks after surgery. 3. Careful observation without further immediate treatment in selected patients. 4. Treatment for patients with urinary problems: radiation, hormones, surgery to treat symptoms, or clinical trials. 5. Clinical trials: radiation seeding, neutron/photon radiation or ultrasound-guided cryosurgery, or other trials.
Stage IV T4a, T4b, N0 M0; any T, N1–3, M0; any T, any N, M1; Stage D1, D2	Cancer cells have spread to lymph nodes or to organs and tissues far away from prostate. T4a means that cancer cells have spread to neck of bladder, sphincter muscle, or rectum. T4b means spread to levator muscles or is attached to pelvic wall. N1–3 indicate cancer has spread to lymph nodes.	Treatment is determined by age, other illnesses, symptoms, spread to bone or lymph nodes. 1. Hormonal treatment: orchiectomy alone or with flutamide or nilutamide; LHRH agonists; leuprolide plus flutamide; estrogens. 2. External radiation (delay 4–6 weeks after a TURP). 3. Radiation to reduce symptoms. 4. Surgery (TURP) to reduce symptoms. 5. Careful observation without further immediate treatment. 6. Clinical trials: neutron/photon radiation; radical prostatectomy plus orchiectomy; chemotherapy; antiandrogens alone or with other hormone treatment.
Recurrent	Cancer has come back after it has been treated. It may come back in the prostate or in another part of the body.	1. Radiation if recurrence is in the prostate area (if prior treatment was prostatectomy). 2. Hormones. 3. Clinical trials: chemotherapy or biologic agents.

T = size of tumor and level of invasion.
N = lymph node involvement, size, number.
M = metastases.

What is the Jewett system of staging?

This system uses the letters A through D to indicate approximately the same categories as the I to IV system. So if your doctor refers to your cancer as a Stage A1, you will understand that it is approximately in the same category as a Stage I.

Does cancer of the prostate sometimes spread?

Cancer cells can break away from the original tumor in the prostate and spread through the bloodstream and lymphatic system and form tumors in other parts of the body. When cancer of the prostate spreads outside the prostate itself, it often shows up in nearby lymph nodes or lymph glands. Prostate cancer can also spread to the bones, liver, lungs, bladder, and other organs. When cancer spreads from the prostate to other parts of the body, often to the bone, the disease is identified as metastatic prostate cancer rather than bone cancer, liver cancer, and so on. Usually, the PSA test is used to determine if there has been spread. To determine if there are other signs of cancer, the doctor may order a CT or CAT scan to check for swollen lymph nodes or an MRI to check the prostate and nearby lymph nodes. A bone scan may be ordered to check the bones since rapid growth of bone lesions may be a sign of spreading cancer, although growth can also result from other bone problems. A chest x-ray may also be done to check the lungs.

chapter 6

Understanding Your Treatment Choices

There are many more possible treatment choices than you might have been led to believe. Some have been used for many years. Others have not been tested fully but are being explored. Many men are deciding to try some of the more experimental methods because they fear the consequences of some of the standard treatments. One thing you should be aware of is that no method is entirely risk free. Some methods have been used for a longer period than others, so the results cover a longer period of time. The biggest problem if you have early-stage prostate cancer is that it is difficult for your doctor to know whether or not your cancer will progress and metastasize. This dilemma is the principal reason for the differences of opinion among doctors.

Even the top physicians in urology cannot agree on which method of treatment is best for prostate cancer. According to the National Cancer Institute, "in a literature review of case series of patients with palpable, clinically localized disease, the authors found that

WHAT TREATMENT DO DOCTORS PREFER?

In 1988 a survey was done of 304 urologists, radiation oncologists, and oncologists in the United States, Canada, and Great Britain. Each one was asked what treatment he would choose if he was 67 years of age, diagnosed with cancer confined to the prostate, and had moderately differentiated prostate cancer. Of the American urologists (whose specialty is surgery), 79 percent said they would have surgery, whereas 92 percent of the radiologists chose radiation. Among the British doctors, 4 percent chose surgery, 44 percent chose radiation, and 52 percent chose watchful waiting. This survey is dated, but it puts the debate in perspective.

10-year prostate cancer-specific survival rates were best in radical prostatectomy series (about 93 percent), worst in radiation therapy series (about 75 percent) and intermediate with deferred treatment (about 85 percent). Since it is highly unlikely that radiation would worsen disease-specific survival, the most likely explanation is that selection factors affect choice of treatment. Such selection factors make comparisons of therapeutic strategies imprecise. Unfortunately, these series constitute the same data on which opinions regarding management of clinically localized cancer are based."

Each method as well as many of the newer and less well-tested treaments has its advantages and disadvantages. What you need to untangle and determine is which method best suits the way you choose to live. Your quality of life is an important factor. Although there are advantages and disadvantages to each treatment, there are treatments available to you to control your cancer even though you may not be totally happy with some of the consequences of some of them.

The most commonly used treatments are:

- **Prostatectomy:** The prostate is completely removed in an operation.
- **External radiation:** A linear accelerator delivers radiation to the area. It is usually given five times a week for seven weeks.

- **Hormonal manipulation:** This involves removal or suppression of the male hormone testosterone. Either a suppressor hormone (Lupron) is injected or the testicles are removed (orchiectomy). It is usually used prior to other treatment for removal of the prostate or when the cancer has advanced.
- **Watchful waiting:** Watchful waiting is used when cancer cannot be felt but is signaled by other testing or for older men who have decided that quality of life is more important than the statistically short time that may be gained through aggressive therapy.

Some other treatments still considered in the testing stage include:

- **Radiation seeding (internal radiation or brachytherapy):** Radioactive seeds are implanted in the prostate.
- **Cryosurgery:** Freezing techniques are used to destroy the prostate.
- **Chemotherapy:** Chemotherapy has not proven to be successful in the past, but a combination of drugs as well as chemotherapy implants are in clinical trials. It is not used for early-stage cancers.
- **Hyperthermia:** A variety of techniques employing heat have been used to treat tumors. Emerging techniques using a variety of methods, including microwaves, are presently being studied in various parts of the world.
- **Other:** Other less conventional and more controversial and experimental approaches, including nutritional therapies, which have not been clinically verified or tested, are being used (see Chapter 14).

QUESTIONS TO ASK BEFORE DECIDING ON ANY TREATMENT FOR PROSTATE CANCER

- What type of treatment do you suggest?
- Why do you feel this treatment is better for me than other possible treatments?
- Are there other treatments that will achieve the same results?

DECISION-MAKING FACTORS

Type of Treatment	Procedure	Pros and Cons
Radical prostatectomy Approaches to surgery listed below are determined by physician, but it is important for you to understand what is being planned.	Removal of entire prostate including seminal vesicles and small cuff of attached bladder neck.	Considered a cure if cancer is localized to the prostate. Lymph nodes removed to determine if it has spread. If spread is detected, many surgeons do not continue with operation. Cost: $15,000–$18,000.
Radical retropubic prostatectomy	Most commonly used method. Open surgery through 6-inch vertical incision in lower abdomen; often possible to preserve nerves that produce erection (see nerve-sparing prostatectomy).	Impotence (60–90%); incontinence (30–60%); difficulty urinating; best for large prostates; allows lymph node dissection for staging; fewer rectal injuries.
Radical perineal prostatectomy	Surgery done through incision between anus and scrotum.	Good choice for heavier men; lymph nodes cannot be removed through same incision. Difficult to do nerve-sparing operation.
Nerve-sparing prostatectomy	Surgery performed with specific aim of preserving erectile function; often only nerve on side opposite cancer is spared to assure all cancer cells removed. Not always possible to spare potency.	Impotence (30–60%); if both nerves spared, may expose patient to risk of leaving cancer cells in area surrounding prostate. Must be done by an expert. Cost: $18,000–$20,000.

External radiation	Machine directs high-energy rays or particles at prostate for a period of weeks.	Possible radiation effects to rectum and bladder. Diarrhea or urinary frequency. Impotence (40%). Potency progressively may diminish. Little incontinence. Some studies show radiation may be comparable to surgery, without side effects of prostatectomy. Cost: $8,000–$12,000 for radiation treatment.
Radiation seeding Internal radiation (brachytherapy)	Radiation seeds are inserted into the prostate either with or without surgery. Use of ultrasound has helped make it possible to implant more accurately. Allows higher dose of radiation directly to prostate. (Lymph node dissection may be done as separate procedure.)	Wide variability of complication rates. Less risk of impotence (25%). Some loss of sexual performance. Little incontinence (0–2%). Cost: $10,000–$15,000 including lymph node dissection.
Watchful waiting	No treatment. An alternative for men, especially those over 70, with localized disease. Must have follow-up PSA, prostate exams, and urinalysis every 6 months.	Tumor may get larger and grow outside prostate. Can decide later to have treatment.

(continued)

DECISION-MAKING FACTORS (cont.)

Type of Treatment	Procedure	Pros and Cons
Cryosurgery	Destruction of tissue by freezing; probe is inserted into tumor. Experimental treatment.	Short hospitalization and recovery period. Frequent urination, burning and pain with urination. High percentage become impotent (80%). Cost: $12,000–$14,000.
Hormone treatment	Pills and or monthly injections of hormones.	Hot flashes, decreased libido, some breast enlargement. Not considered curative. Cost: $400–$600 monthly.
Orchiectomy	Surgery to remove testicles to eliminate major source of testosterone.	Hot flashes, decreased libido. Not considered curative. Cost: $2,000–$3,000.
Hyperthermia	Heating with a probe raises temperatures 20–40% above normal body temperature to destroy prostate tissue. At this time, an experimental method.	Though various types of hyperthermia have been used over the last century without definitive results, emerging techniques are being studied.

Chemotherapy	Variety of cancer drugs, such as lovastatin, strontium, CPT-11, interferon, ketoconazole, suramin, topotecan, retinoids, and taxol, being tested in clinical trials.	Numerous drugs being tried on metastatic or recurrent cancer in clinical trials. Costs depend upon drug and how administered.
Lymph node dissection	Done for diagnostic purposes. Sometimes done with a laparoscope as separate operation (through 4 small incisions) to determine if cancer has spread before radiation or other treatment.	If done with prostatectomy, it is part of the operation. May impair lymphatic drainage, causing lymphedema. Lymphedema may occur years after primary treatment. Cost of laparoscopic lymphandectomy: $2,500–$4,000.
Laser surgery	Done with laser. May be used when patient has radiation and blockage needs to be opened up.	Not considered a primary treatment at this time. Does not cause bleeding; fewer risks of immediate surgical complications. Requires catheter for longer period. Longer recovery. No tissue available for biopsy.

- Is it possible for me to have no treatment at this time but to have you follow me closely to see if there are future changes?
- What are the benefits and drawbacks of each kind of treatment?
- What are the drawbacks to having radiation instead of surgery or surgery instead of radiation?
- Is radiation seeding a possibility for my condition?
- Will radiation be used following surgery?
- How often do you do this type of surgery or radiation?
- Can I have radiation (either internal or external) and later, if it doesn't work, have surgery or cryosurgery? Is it worth the risk?
- How extensive will the surgery or radiation be?
- Where will the scar be?
- Can you do nerve-sparing surgery so that I will not be impotent? How successful has this surgery been in your patients to date?
- Is cryosurgery a possibility?
- Do you recommend hyperthermia?
- What about hormonal treatment?
- How will the treatment affect my sex life?
- If I lose my ability to function sexually, what do you suggest for alternatives?
- Will treatment make me incontinent? How long will incontinence continue? Will incontinence be permanent? Can exercises help me alleviate incontinence?
- Will you be doing extensive lymph node dissection to check for cancer spread? Will doing the dissection change your treatment plans? What are the side effects in your experience?
- What restrictions will there be on my activities after treatment?
- When can I return to normal activities after this treatment?

Does age make a difference in deciding what kind of treatment option to choose for prostate cancer?

Since prostate cancer is slow growing, many doctors feel that a 70- to 75-year-old man diagnosed with an early stage of prostate cancer should probably opt for the least invasive treatment. Watchful waiting may be the answer for some. Hormonal treatment or radiation might be recommended for others rather than surgery, since they have fewer side effects. In younger or more active men, the decision is less clear: surgery to remove the entire prostate may be recommended. You should be aware that there is a great deal of controversy about what treatment is best and at what age it is wise to opt for less invasive treatment. Although some early results are in, most studies are incomplete as to how the effectiveness of each of the treatments compare in long-term results.

What does the National Cancer Institute say about how to treat localized prostate cancer?

The National Cancer Institute has noted that much of the data that are being used to make treatment decisions are not comparable, and therefore, comparisons of the different choices of treatments are imprecise.

Are there any studies that assess watchful waiting as a treatment?

There is a study being carried out by the National Cancer Institute, the Department of Veterans Affairs, and the Agency for Health Care Policy and Research called the PIVOT trial. It is enrolling about 2,000 men over a several-year period and following them for up to 15 years. The men will be divided randomly into two groups. One-half will have a radical prostatectomy and the other half will have watchful waiting—being closely followed by physicians with PSA, digital, and other exams. Unfortunately, it will be many years before we get the answer from this clinical trial. One other study that compared these two alternatives showed no significant differences in survival, but it was too small and did not include other information needed to make general conclusions.

Are there differences of opinion on how severe the side effects are from the different treatments?

There are wide variations on the estimates of how often side effects are seen and how they impact men's lives. Patient surveys show that side effects, especially those such as impotence and incontinence, occur more often than what has been estimated by

COMPARING SIDE EFFECTS OF MOST COMMONLY USED TREATMENTS

	IMPOTENCE	INCONTINENCE	DIFFICULT URINATION	RECTAL PROBLEMS	FURTHER TREATMENT
Surgery	60–90%; 30–50% if nerves are spared	20–30% have some long-term incontinence; 5–7% have severe incontinence	12–20%	3%	30–65% have follow-up radiation
Radiation	About 40% over long term	6% have some long-term; 7% have severe incontinence	5%	11%	No information
Radiation Seeding	25%	0–2%; 15% if treatment given after TURP		20%	No information
Cryo-surgery	70–80%; it is believed these figures may improve as techniques improve; erection ability may return over time	10%; this figure rises to 50–70% in men who had prior radiation	Blocked urethra, 10–30%		No information

doctors or usually reported in the medical literature, and may be dependent upon who is giving the treatment to you.

Before going any further, assess your own priorities on these key issues:

- How important is it to me to know the cancer has been removed regardless of the consequences?
- How important is it to me to avoid being incontinent?
- How important is it to me to preserve my ability to have an erection?

---

chapter 7

Getting Other Opinions

Your diagnosis is in. You've taken all the tests and checked basic information about your prostate problems and it looks like you are dealing with cancer. Suppose, however, you're not absolutely comfortable with going ahead with the treatment the doctor has recommended for you. Or perhaps you feel that you'd like to have some confirmation of the diagnosis. Or you may have decided that you want to look further before making a decision. It's a good idea to check out your own feelings before drawing any conclusions. You need to understand the possible avenues before you make a definite choice. There are many: searching for additional information, getting a second opinion, or even changing doctors.

QUESTIONS TO ASK YOURSELF BEFORE MAKING ANY DECISIONS

- Have I gotten full information from the doctor about my cancer—stage, grade, type, and so on?

- Am I prepared to accept the fact that the treatment may leave me incontinent, impotent, or both?
- Have I discussed the pros and cons with my partner?
- What are the side effects of other types of treatment?
- Do I want to get another opinion before proceeding with the treatment this doctor recommends?
- Do I want to get a second opinion from a surgeon if I originally saw a radiation oncologist or see a radiation oncologist if I saw a surgeon?
- Do I want to explore other treatment possibilities such as cryosurgery or watchful waiting?

How can I take get information on different kinds of treatments, including experimental treatment?

You can call the National Cancer Institute's Cancer Information Service, a toll-free telephone number (1-800-4-CANCER). The National Cancer Institute is the federal government's principal agency for research on cancer prevention, diagnosis, treatment, and rehabilitation. Trained information specialists can tell you the kinds of treatments available for your specific type and stage of prostate cancer and, if appropriate, can conduct a PDQ search for those treatments in clinical trials and where they are being conducted.

What is PDQ?

PDQ (Protocol Data Query) is a computerized database that gives information on the state-of-the-art treatment for each type and stage of most cancers as well as information on more than 1,000 active investigational or experimental treatment studies underway in the United States. If you want to have a PDQ search done, you will need to know the cell type of your cancer, the stage of disease, the kinds of treatments you have already had, and when you had them. All the material you get from the Cancer Information Service is free. It is a good place to start your search for information.

EXPLORING YOUR THOUGHTS ABOUT TREATMENT CHOICES

NOTE YOUR FEELINGS HERE	QUESTION	COMMENTS
	Do I want to check how different treatments might affect my life?	Different treatments have specific side effects. You may find it helpful to check out expected side effects before making a decision. In addition to the standard treatments, there are some experimental treatments you may want to explore.
	Is it true that I have plenty of time to make a decision?	This is a decision that does not need to be rushed—most prostate cancers are slow growing and a few extra weeks, or even months, to check out choices usually will not make a difference in the long term.
	Am I one of those men who just want to know that the cancer has been removed so I don't have to think about it again?	If you are, you should be aware that it is not always possible to remove all of the cancer or to be certain that it has not already spread. Study the pros and cons and probe your own feelings to determine if just "knowing" that the cancer has been removed will honestly relieve you of worry.

If the prostate is removed for BPH, does that mean I can't get cancer?	Some men think that surgery for BPH, which consists of removing part of the middle of the prostate, means that they do not have to worry about cancer. However, the remaining prostate tissue can become cancerous. Even the removal of the entire prostate does not always guarantee that the cancer has been completely removed from the body.
Is it true that at 70 years of age, treatment for prostate cancer is known to extend life by only 1 to 6 months?	That's what statistics presently show. This is the reason why many doctors recommend watchful waiting as the treatment of choice for many men over 70.
How often do men become impotent from having a prostatectomy?	For a normal prostatectomy, 60 to 90 out of 100 men become impotent; for those who are able to have nerve-sparing surgery, 30 to 50 out of 100.
How often do men become impotent from external radiation for prostate cancer?	From 40 to 65 of each 100 men who have external radiation become impotent over time.

(continued)

EXPLORING YOUR THOUGHTS ABOUT TREATMENT CHOICES *(cont.)*

NOTE YOUR FEELINGS HERE	QUESTION	COMMENTS
	How often do men become impotent following radiation seeding?	Early results show that for those who have radiation seeding, impotence can be expected in 25% of those under 70 years of age. The number rises to 50% for those over 70. This treatment is still in clinical trials.
	How often do men become impotent following cryosurgery?	Seventy to 80 of each 100 men who have cryosurgery can expect to become impotent, although there is some early evidence that recovery of erection is possible. This treatment is still in clinical trials.
	How often do men become incontinent after prostate cancer treatment?	Immediately after **surgery**, all men are incontinent. About 20–30 of 100 men who have prostatectomy report some ongoing incontinence and the need to wear pads; 7 of 100 men report severe incontinence after 2 to 4 years. Six of every 100 who have **external radiation** report incontinence. **Radiation seeding** does not usually cause incontinence if there has not been prior urinary tract surgery. **Cryosurgery** incontinence to date is reported at 1 or 2 in 100, rising to 50% in men who have had prior radiation.

What percentage of men need radiation after prostate surgery?	Sixty-five of 100 men who have a prostatectomy will need to have radiation treatment after surgery.
What are the risks of cryosurgery?	The risks appear to be similar to those of any surgical procedure, though there seem to be fewer incidences of major complications, a shortened hospital stay, and the ability to have the procedure repeated if necessary.
Is hormonal therapy an option?	Hormonal therapy is being used in a number of different ways, some of which are untested. When used for cases where cancer has metastasized to the bones, it can prolong survival from 3 to 10 years. Hormonal therapy is done either with drugs or with the removal of the testicles, which causes impotence. It is sometimes used to reduce the size of the cancer before other treatment.

(continued)

EXPLORING YOUR THOUGHTS ABOUT TREATMENT CHOICES *(cont.)*

NOTE YOUR FEELINGS HERE	QUESTION	COMMENTS
	Is watchful waiting a wise option?	It depends on your age, general health, family history, and the size and type of cancer you have. You are betting that you will probably die of something else before the prostate cancer becomes a problem. Regular monitoring is a must.
	Is chemotherapy being used to treat prostate cancer?	Most chemotherapy drugs have not worked well as the main treatment. However, some advanced prostate cancers are now being treated with chemotherapy in clinical trials. Side effects will depend upon type of drugs used. May include nausea, vomiting, hair loss, etc.
	Does the stage of cancer you have determine what treatment is best?	Yes, so it is important for you to know the stage of your cancer as well as your Gleason grade when you are weighing your options.

How would I go about doing my search for additional information on treatment options?

A reference librarian in a good-sized library is a good person to start with. If there is a medical library nearby, it is worth a visit, because it will have a broad selection of information and a wide selection of medical journals. Talk to the reference librarian about what it is that you are seeking. Make sure that any book you are looking at is recently published, because there is new information coming out almost daily. The reference librarian can help you do a search of journal articles; the *Index Medicus* refers you to articles in medical and related health-science journals. Ask if there is a fee and how much it is.

Aren't medical publications difficult to read?

Yes, they are. But the first section of each medical article, called an abstract, is usually an overview of the article's contents and any conclusions that have been made. This section along with the discussion and conclusion area of the article are usually the easiest to read. You need to understand that the articles are the opinions of the authors; read several articles to get differing views. It is also useful to discuss any information with your doctor, who can help interpret the materials and clear up any concerns you might have about it.

Can I do a search on my own computer?

Yes. There is lots of health advice being given through the Internet or with one of the major on-line services—CompuServe, Prodigy, and America Online. There are forums, chat areas, on-line medical clinics, bulletin boards, and message boards. Some of the information is quite useful and from very legitimate, authorized sources (both the National Cancer Institute and the American Cancer Society have information on-line). You need to understand that there are no built-in controls or restrictions to regulate the kind of information that is being given. Some of the information on-line is from marketing and selling enterprises trying to sell their products. Others are patients who are sharing their experiences. Be sure you look at the source of what is being presented. Most on-line services tell you that you are taking the advice at your own risk.

How do I reach some of the health on-line services?

If you can access the Internet with the World Wide Web, here are some addresses to start with:

- National Cancer Institute: http://wwwicic.nci.nih.gov/
- American Cancer Society: http://www.cancer.org
- Prostate Cancer Home Page://www.cancer.med.umich.edu/ prostcan/prostcan.htm/
- Prostate Cancer Infoline: http://www.comed.com/Prostate

You can also access health information on other services (see Chapter 16).

How can I check to make sure the information I am getting from these on-line sources is legitimate?

You need to be a good consumer. If the information is from health professionals, check their credentials. If articles are mentioned, look for them and read them. See what kind of publication they are in. If someone is claiming miraculous results, look closely at the science behind them. Be alert to those who say that the medical community is not listening to them and who promise more than can possibly be delivered (see Chapter 14).

What kind of doctor should I go to for another opinion?

It depends on what kind of doctor you have already talked with. Understanding what different doctors' specialties are is helpful. Urologists treat the prostate as well as the rest of the urinary system, including kidneys, bladder, adrenal glands, and testes. The radiation oncologist uses radiation in the treatment of cancer; the diagnostic radiologist uses x-rays, computerized tomographic scans, and magnetic resonance images for diagnosis of cancer. An oncologist is a doctor who deals exclusively with cancer patients. If you are planning on having surgery, look for a cancer surgeon who is certified by the American Board of Surgeons in Urologic Surgery. If you are considering one of the newer treatments, such as cryosurgery or radiation seeding, you need to seek out a specialist who has experience with these procedures.

How do I go about getting another opinion?

- You can ask your primary doctor to suggest the names of urologists, radiation oncologists, or specialists to see for a second opinion.
- You can make the appointment yourself, or you can ask the doctor to make the appointment for you.
- You should always discuss your plans for consultation with your doctor. You will need to bring your original x-rays and tests for the other doctor to use during your consultation. If your doctor is uncooperative, then you have other decisions to make about continuing that relationship.
- If possible, it is best to get your second opinion outside the particular group where your primary doctor is located.
- You can call your nearest medical school and ask for suggestions. A medical school's outpatient clinic, where some of the country's top specialists practice, is also a good place to check.
- You can call the American Board of Certified Specialties at 1-800-776-CERT for names of specialists in your area.
- You can check *The Directory of Medical Specialists* at your library and call the specialist directly.
- You can check *The Directory of Medical Specialists* to get the names of two or three doctors in your area, and ask your doctor to suggest which one you should see.
- Some hospitals have a special telephone line for physician referral, although many simply give names of all the doctors who have privileges to admit patients to their facilities. You also can write the director of the hospital of your choice and ask for suggestions.

Why should I consider getting a second opinion?

There are several reasons for wanting to get a second and possibly a third opinion from another qualified physician. Foremost is reassurance that the first opinion is correct and that you have explored all your choices. Especially in the case of a diagnosis of prostate cancer, a further opinion is a good idea because it will allow you the opportunity to discuss the different possibilities with a doctor from a different discipline. Because there is no full consensus among physicians on which treatment is best for prostate cancer, it becomes really important for you to determine which treatment is best for your particular situation. Getting opinions from doctors in other specialties is a good way to start formulating your own pros and cons on which treatment to have.

Won't my doctor be offended if I ask for another opinion?

If your doctor is offended, then you have a good reason for finding another doctor. The important point to remember is that most doctors *welcome* a second opinion. A second opinion does not mean you are questioning your doctor's competence. If you have cancer, a decision about how you proceed with treatment is among the most important decisions you will make in your life. You need the best advice you can get before proceeding with a course of treatment. You don't hesitate to check out various makes and models of cars when you are buying. You should not hesitate to check out all the possible angles before making a decision about your health and your future. **Remember, the choices you make at the very beginning are the most important ones.**

How can I tell my doctor I want another opinion?

You can simply explain to your doctor that before going any further you would like to talk with someone else. This is not an unusual or unreasonable request. It is a very necessary step for you to take. The doctor may tell you that the tests are conclusive. Do not let that put you off or pressure you into backing down. Explain again that you want another opinion and would like to explore various options. You can say that doing this will help you strengthen the recommendations the doctor has made and will set your mind at ease.

Is a medical school a good place to go for a second opinion?

This is an excellent place to turn for a second opinion. Physicians who practice there are on the faculty of the medical school and are usually using the latest methods of treatment. Because most departments are divided into specialties, this is where some of the top specialists in the country practice. You can contact the clinic by calling the medical school and explaining that you are interested in contacting a doctor who specializes in the area of your specific problem. Don't be afraid to explain that you want to get a second opinion and to describe your experience to date. Each department, of course, has its own setup, but most have appointment secretaries who are very knowledgeable about the service and the doctors in it and will be most helpful in making arrangements for a consultation.

How do I get an appointment for a consultation?

Sometimes the doctor who refers you will make the appointment for you. If you are calling yourself, explain that you have already had a diagnosis and wish to make an appointment for a consultation. Don't make the mistake of trying to let the doctor think you haven't been to another doctor. Using a specialist on a consulting basis means that you will get a straight answer, since that doctor has nothing to gain from recommending one treatment over another.

Does having a consultation at a medical school mean I have to go there for treatment?

You have free choice in the matter. The decision is yours. Sometimes people shy away from getting expert advice from doctors at a large medical center because they feel this will mean that they have to return there for treatments. Many medical and cancer centers diagnose and recommend treatment for patients to be followed by doctors in local communities. If the medical center is a long distance from your home and you do not want the expense and inconvenience of returning there each time you need treatment, you can take advantage of a consultation and continue to be treated by your own doctor and at your local hospital.

What is the difference between a referral and a consultation?

If your doctor decides that you require the attention of a specialist, you will probably be given the names of one or several specialists for you to see. This is called a referral and differs from a consultation. A referral means that once you see the specialist you become that doctor's patient. In a consultation, the consulting doctor advises you but does not take over responsibility for treating you unless you personally decide you wish to change doctors.

Who pays for a second opinion?

Many insurance companies now pay for second opinions. Some even require them. Even if your particular insurance company does not pay, the cost of a consultation is considerably less than the first opinion because all the test results and x-rays are already available to the second doctor.

What will a consultation or second opinion cost?

You will be amazed to find that some of the finest physicians in the country charge no more—and sometimes considerably less— than doctors with far less experience and expertise. Part of the reason is that medical school faculty physicians are often salaried and their fees are returned to the medical school.

Is it appropriate for me to take notes or tape-record my conversation with the doctor?

It is perfectly acceptable for patients to take notes or even ask to record discussions with physicians. However, it is best to mention to your doctor that you plan to tape the information. Explain that you want to use it as a refresher when you get home rather than having to call back to ask the doctor to repeat the information for you or your family members. Some doctors, concerned about malpractice suits, may not be entirely comfortable with this, but a taped record can be very helpful to you in reviewing a consultation or it can be used to get feedback from someone who is not present during the appointment.

What if I decide I want to change doctors?

This is more difficult than asking for another opinion. If you are not satisfied with your relationship with your doctor, you have every right to choose another doctor. Whatever your reason for wanting to change—whether it is because you want someone with more experience to treat you, you have lost confidence in the ability of your present doctor to treat you, or you wish to make the change for personality reasons—if you are feeling negative about your doctor, it is not in your best interests to continue the relationship. You should not be afraid to be honest with your doctor about wanting to change. No doctor likes to lose a patient, but every doctor has had that experience.

You might handle the discussion diplomatically by thanking your doctor for what has been done, assuring the doctor that you appreciate all the help that has been given to you, but that you would prefer to try to find another doctor who is more suitable for your particular needs at this time. Your doctor is legally obligated to provide your new doctor with any existing records, x-rays, and test results.

How can I find a new doctor who specializes in prostate cancer?

This can work in a number of ways. You can talk to friends who are nurses or doctors for references. You can call the local chapter of the American Cancer Society. You can call a medical school or a cancer center for information. You might want to discuss the results of your own research for a specialist with your primary doctor, who will usually want to make a recommendation. Sometimes your primary doctor will give you more than one name. You should be sure to determine the specialist's credentials and be sure you have the answers to these questions:

- Why are you referring me to this particular doctor?
- Is this doctor a specialist in doing this procedure (or in this field)?
- How often does this specialist perform the particular operation (or service)?
- Is the doctor board certified? On the staff of an accredited hospital?

Why is it important that the doctor be board certified?

The doctor who is board certified meets very rigid requirements. For instance, a urologist must provide a detailed account of every surgery performed for at least 12 months. If the list is approved, the doctor is required to take an exhaustive two-day written and oral exam. The doctor is certified if all parts of the exam are passed. Urologists who were first board certified in the mid-1980s or later are required to retake the certification exam every 10 years to maintain board certification. Urologists who were board certified before the mid-1980s are not required to be retested.

Will I be able to have another opinion on treatment if I belong to an HMO (health maintenance organization) or insurance plan?

Most HMOs or insurance plans have contracted urology specialists for referrals. If the urologist in the HMO is not to your liking, you may decide to go outside the HMO network. Be sure you understand what it will cost you if you decide to have a second opinion or wish to be treated outside the network. You need to find out if your plan has an opt-out or point-of-service feature where the employer pays some of the cost, usually 60 to 70 percent, if you obtain care outside the HMO. If possible, you may want to check with someone in the plan with a similar condition to see how things worked out.

Does Medicare cover the cost of prostate cancer treatment?

Many of the treatments for prostate cancer are covered by Medicare. Medicare Hospital Insurance, Part A, covers room and board in a semiprivate room, nursing care, supplies and equipment, x-ray, radiology, operating room, medical supplies, and lab tests. Part B, which must be applied for separately and is an optional plan, covers 80 percent of the allowable charges. It is intended to fill some of the gaps left in medical insurance coverage under Part A. The major benefit under Part B is payment for physician's services. Covered by Part B are: medical and surgical services of the physician in the hospital, nursing home, office, clinic, or patient's home. It covers radiology and pathology costs as well as services prescribed by the physician in connection with diagnosis and treatment. Cryosurgery and some of the other treatments still considered experimental are not always covered. Be sure to check before you have the treatment to find out what your coverage will be.

What should I know about the billing balance?

If your physician is a participating physician (one who has agreed to accept the charges established by Medicare), the doctor will be paid 80 percent of the established charge. You will pay the other 20 percent. If you have Medigap insurance, it will usually cover the 20 percent. Be sure you are not confused by the billing balance that some physicians who are not participating physicians add to your copayment bill. For instance, if Medicare pays $100 as a reasonable charge, a nonparticipating physician may charge $120 for the procedure. Medicare would pay the patient or physician $80. If you pay the $20 copayment, $20 will remain as the billing balance. If your state has legislated against the practice of balance billing, you are not responsible for that balance.

chapter 8

What Happens If I Have My Prostate Removed by Surgery?

> Prostate surgery, called a *prostatectomy*, is commonly used to treat cancer of the prostate. Many men still believe that they want to have the cancer taken out and make the decision that the best method for them is by surgical removal of the prostate. The possible fallacy in this approach is that surgery may *not* get it all out. The cancer may have spread even though it is not visible. Statistics indicate that about half of the men who have a radical prostatectomy need to have additional treatment within five years of the operation.

Since the PSA test began to be commonly used (figures are available for 1984 to 1990), the rate of radical prostatectomies increased by 575 percent. In 1990, more radical prostatectomies were performed on Medicare patients than in the three years between 1984 and 1986. Between 1991 and 1993, the number of radical prostatectomies soared from 50,000 to 100,000. Some research seems to indicate that a 70-year-old man with localized

prostate cancer who had surgery or radiation treatment would live
only four to six months longer than one who did not have treatment.

There is a great difference in the rate of prostatectomies performed in different parts of the country. In 1989, for example,
the probability that a 65-year-old man would have a radical prostatectomy during the next 10 years was just over 1 percent. In
Seattle, the rate was close to 6 percent.

Before getting involved with any treatment, you should know
exactly what you are getting into. This is especially true with prostate surgery, which includes the surgical removal of the prostate
gland and the seminal vesicles. In performing the operation, the
surgeon brings the bladder down to the pelvis, and the bladder
neck is attached to the remaining urethra where the prostate
gland originally was attached. In addition, lymph nodes are removed to check if the cancer has spread. This is a major operation, and its consequences need to be understood.

Long-term problems that can be expected after surgery in a
group of 100 men who had prostate surgery include:

Impotence	60–90
Impotence after nerve-sparing surgery	30–50
Some long-term incontinence	20–30
Severe incontinence	5–7
Difficult urination	12–20
Rectal injury	3
Follow-up radiation	45–65

Here are some facts to take into consideration in making your
decision:

• **Younger men who have no serious illness are usually advised to consider surgery if the cancer is confined to the
prostate. For these men with a long life expectancy, surgery may be the best treatment choice. However, there is
some controversy among experts about this assumption,
because some contend that radiation treatment is a comparable alternative. In older men, risks and complications associated with surgery increase and may outweigh benefits.**

- The major published results of the success of radical prostatectomy come from a few centers that are known for
surgical excellence. So if you are planning to have a prostatectomy, choose your surgeon and hospital carefully.
- It is important that your surgeon or urologist performs the
prostatectomy procedure daily or at least weekly. There is
the question of whether someone who performs the procedure occasionally can do it with the same success as someone who performs it on a regular basis. It is best to have a
urologist who is board certified.
- It is difficult to compare prostatectomy results done in
hospitals outside the major medical centers, because most
studies are done in major centers and the treatment results of most community practitioners usually are not analyzed or included in the studies published in the medical
literature.

QUESTIONS TO ASK YOUR DOCTOR BEFORE HAVING PROSTATE SURGERY

- What kinds of operation will you be doing?
- What do you consider the advantages of surgery over
other treatments for my prostate cancer?
- Will you do nerve-sparing surgery? How successful has it
been in your experience?
- What are my chances of becoming impotent? Will this be
temporary or permanent?
- What sort of limitations will the operation put on my sex-
ual activity?
- What percentage of your patients are permanently inconti-
nent?
- Will you be doing retropubic or perineal surgery?
- Where will the scar be?
- What kinds of tests will I need before my operation?
- Would it be appropriate for me to have hormone therapy
before surgery to reduce the size of the tumor?
- Should I plan to bank my blood beforehand in case a
transfusion is needed?

- What kind of anesthesia will be used? Epidural? Spinal? What are the advantages of each?
- How long does the operation take?
- Will I have drains, catheters, and intravenous lines after my operation?
- Will I need a nurse when I come out of surgery?
- How soon will I be up out of bed?
- Does the hospital have patient-controlled painkiller equipment so I can control how much painkiller I receive?
- Is it your practice to check the lymph nodes first with a lymphadenectomy before proceeding with the removal of the prostate?
- What happens if you find the cancer has spread?
- What is the possibility that I will need additional treatment following surgery?
- How long will I be in the hospital?

What is a prostatectomy?

A prostatectomy is the surgical removal of all or part of the prostate. A radical or total prostatectomy is the removal of the **entire** prostate. A radical prostatectomy is the surgery used for treating prostate cancer.

Is prostate removal surgery ever done on an outpatient basis?

There are a few centers where prostate surgery is being done with an overnight or two-night hospital stay. Usually epidural anesthesia is used instead of general anesthesia and postoperative narcotics are replaced with less complex pain relievers.

What are the chances of my being incontinent and impotent following surgery?

Much depends on the location of the cancer and the skill of the surgeon. If the cancer has spread outside the prostate capsule, the surgeon performing the prostatectomy may have to cut the nerves that control erection. Additionally, the skill of the surgeon and the location of the tumor have a great deal to do with the outcome. According to the National Cancer Institute, among men over 65 years of age, 60 to 90 percent of men who have had prostate cancer surgery are impotent following surgery. All men who have had prostate surgery are incontinent for the first few weeks. The amount of time men remain incontinent varies greatly—for many it can take up to a year. About 20 to 30 percent of men have some kind of long-term incontinence. It is important to question the doctor carefully about his experience and the results achieved with patients, because studies show that results differ substantially from doctor to doctor.

Is hormone therapy ever used before surgery?

Hormone therapy is sometimes prescribed for a number of months before surgery to reduce prostate size or, as doctors say, to "debulk" the tumor.

Will I need other treatments after I have my radical prostatectomy?

A recent study shows that about one out of every three men has had additional treatment within five years of having a radical prostatectomy. The researchers, who studied the Medicare records of over 3,000 men who had radical prostatectomies between 1985 and 1992, found that one out of every three men had radiation therapy, orchiectomy, or hormone therapy within five years of his original surgery. The rate varied, depending upon the tumor grade and the stage of the prostate cancer—only 15 percent of men who had well-differentiated, earlier stage disease received the additional treatment in contrast to nearly 70 percent of those with poorly differentiated, later stage prostate cancer. Since some of the men in this study were diagnosed before the PSA test became available in 1989, these statistics may change as prostate cancer is diagnosed at an earlier stage.

Are there different kinds of prostatectomy operations?

A prostatectomy is done in one of two ways. In a retropubic prostatectomy, the prostate and nearby lymph nodes are removed through an incision in the abdomen. This is the most common method. In a perineal prostatectomy, the incision is made between the scrotum and the anus. Nearby lymph nodes sometimes are removed through a separate incision in the abdomen. It is important to ask your doctor exactly what kind of operation is planned.

What determines which type of prostatectomy operation will be done?

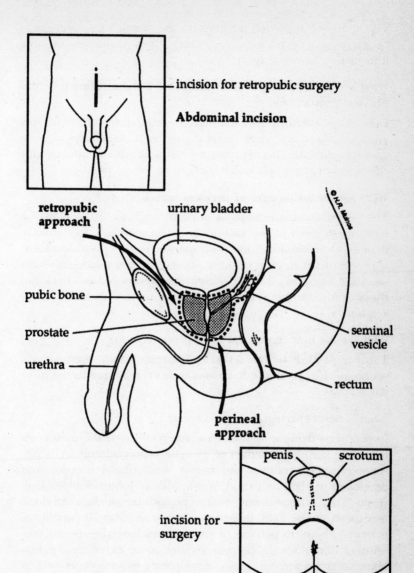

incision for retropubic surgery

Abdominal incision

retropubic
approach

urinary bladder

pubic bone

prostate

urethra

seminal
vesicle

rectum

perineal
approach

penis   scrotum

incision for
surgery

anus

Perineal incision

The choice of approach depends on the doctor's training, surgical expertise, and personal preference. But you should have this information before surgery.

What are the advantages of a retropubic prostatectomy over the perineal prostatectomy?

Doctors who perform this abdominal operation feel that with this approach there are fewer rectal injuries and lower rates of postoperative incontinence. Furthermore, it is possible to operate and check the pelvic lymph nodes without an extra operation.

What are the advantages of perineal prostatectomy?

The perineal prostatectomy is done through an incision in the scrotum, in front of the rectum. It is less traumatic to the body than an abdominal incision, with quicker recovery and less pain. It is often used in men who are obese. The two major disadvantages are that a separate operation may be needed to check the lymph nodes, and it is difficult to spare the nerves that control erection.

Who are the best candidates for a prostatectomy?

Those most likely to have a successful prostatectomy are relatively young, healthy men who have small cancers confined to the prostate.

What is nerve-sparing prostate surgery?

Impotence—being unable to have an erection—is the most common long-lasting side effect of prostate cancer surgery. A nerve-sparing procedure to retain nerves that control erection was developed in 1982 by Patrick Walsh, MD, of Johns Hopkins University. Many surgeons now use this procedure, which, when done by experts in the field, preserves potency in 50 to 70 percent of patients. About 75 percent of patients can have the special procedure. The other 25 percent require more extensive surgery. Many surgeons are doing the nerve-sparing procedure as long as it does not compromise the cancer treatment—something that cannot be determined until the surgery is being performed. Some are now sparing only the nerves on the side of the prostate opposite where the cancer is, rather than both nerves. It is wise to

TYPE OF OPERATION FOR PROSTATE CANCER	PROCEDURE	ADVANTAGES AND DISADVANTAGES
Retropubic prostatectomy	Vertical incision from navel to pubic bone. Prostate, seminal vesicles, and lymph nodes removed through incision in abdomen. Most common operation for prostate cancer.	Fewer rectal injuries and lower rates of incontinence. Not necessary to do separate operation on pelvic lymph nodes because they can be removed through same incision.
Perineal prostatectomy	Incision is made between scrotum and anus. Incision is usually an inverted U around inner side of anus.	Less traumatic surgery, less pain, quicker recovery. Often used on obese men. However, separate operation may be needed to check lymph nodes. May be more difficult to spare nerves that control erection.

ask your surgeon about how he performs the procedure so that you can understand what the aftereffects of your operation will be.

What happens if all the nerves that control erection are removed?

If all the nerves that govern an erection must be removed, then you must face the fact that you will be sexually impotent. Even though you will continue to have the same desires and you can still have an orgasm, you will not be able to become erect. This is a question that you should discuss with your partner as well as with your doctor beforehand. Whatever the outcome, it is helpful to be open about your concerns and discuss them with your partner.

Will I be sterile after a total prostatectomy?

Because the prostate gland produces most of the fluid released at the time of sexual intercourse and climax, patients are sterile—

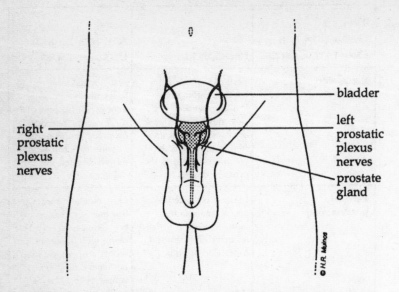

right
prostatic
plexus
nerves

bladder

left
prostatic
plexus
nerves

prostate
gland

© H.R. Malinos

Nerves responsible for erection, found along both sides of the prostate, can be damaged or cut during prostate removal. Nerve-sparing surgery tries to preserve one or both bundles of nerves.

unable to father a child in the normal fashion—following this operation. Removal of the entire prostate gland, including the prostatic urethra, means there is no place for the sperm to be deposited since the vas deferens is divided.

Why is a biopsy done during surgery?

The biopsy is done during surgery to determine whether the cancer has spread beyond the margins or outer edges of the prostate, which may mean that further treatment will be needed (see Chapter 3).

Why is pelvic lymph node dissection (lymphadenectomy) done and why is it important?

Pelvic lymph node dissection is done to determine if the cancer has spread to the lymph nodes since prostate cancer spreads by way of the blood vessels and lymph system. If the lymph nodes

"It was really just a fluke that brought me to the doctor's office," reports Hugh W. "I had retired at 62, had recently moved into a retirement condominium in a new town, and decided I wanted to check out the local doctors. I made an appointment for a physical with the geriatric physician recommended by one of my neighbors. I thought I was in tip-top shape. Even though I'd had blood pressure problems over the years, I was a runner and lately I'd been watching my diet carefully. I was shocked when the doctor said I had an extremely enlarged prostate. I had no symptoms. A few days later, the doctor called to say he'd made an appointment for me with a urologist because my blood tests indicated I had an extremely high PSA—off the charts. The figure I was given was 65. Being totally ignorant of the meaning of the numbers, I was surprised when the urologist told me I would have to come in immediately for a total prostatectomy.

"I decided to do my own investigating. The hospital was a small-town hospital, so I did some research and made appointments at a large cancer center that was within driving distance. Here again, the physicians were startled by my high PSA but did some further testing—biopsies and bone scans—to determine the extent of disease. The biopsies showed that I did have cancer. The bone scans showed no sign of spread. I was given the option of having either radiation therapy or surgery.

"Since I thought getting rid of the cancer was the best way to stop it, I decided to get another opinion concerning surgery from one of the top cancer centers in the country. This time, I went with many questions about the results I could expect as far as incontinence and impotency were concerned. I was told that there was a 50 percent chance that neither of these would happen, especially since my health was so good. And so I went in for surgery. Before the surgery, the doctor told me that if he found any spread of cancer, they would not remove the prostate. I would be closed up and would then have to find another solution to my problem. As it turned out, the cancer had not spread, so the prostatectomy was performed—very successfully, according to the physician. For me, it was not so successful. Two years later, I am unable to have an erection, am still wearing diaper pads, and I'm very angry at the outcome. I feel that the doctor did not give me an honest assessment of the reality of the side effects. If I had to do it over again, I would have had some other type of treatment."

are free of any signs of cancer, this is considered to be proof that the cancer has not spread. The determining factor when deciding whether lymph node dissection is necessary is whether the treatment will be altered if the lymph nodes are found to be cancerous. Physicians do not agree about how extensive dissection of the lymph nodes needs to be, though most physicians are using modified dissection. In a retropubic prostatectomy, lymph node dissection is usually done as a matter of course. Experts feel that in cases where a perineal prostatectomy is being performed, the PSA is below 20, the Gleason score is low grade, and the tumor cannot be felt but was found with ultrasound, the lymph node dissection may be omitted. With larger, less differentiated tumors, a pelvic lymph node dissection is more important.

When is a lymphadenectomy performed?

It depends on the procedure being used. Usually this surgery is performed at the start of a retropubic prostatectomy through a six-inch vertical lower abdominal incision. A pathologist examines the nodes before the surgeon proceeds with the prostatectomy. If no evidence of cancer is found in the lymph nodes, the prostate will be removed. If the nodes are found to be cancerous, surgery will usually be done to remove obstructive tissue, but usually the entire prostate will not be removed.

Is lymphadenectomy ever done ahead of time to determine if there is cancer spread?

A laparoscopic lymphadenectomy is sometimes done when other indicators, such as a high PSA level and a high Gleason score, show there is a possibility of spread. A laparoscopic lymphadenectomy may also be used when a perineal prostatectomy is planned or when another type of treatment has been chosen but the man wishes to have the lymph nodes checked to determine if there has been any spread of the cancer. The laparoscopic procedure for lymph node dissection uses four punctures of about one-half inch each rather than a single incision and takes two to three hours to perform.

What preparation is necessary before prostate surgery?

Preparation is similar to that for most abdominal surgery. Daily enemas and laxatives may be given to remove fecal material so there is a "clean field" for the surgery. The day before surgery you will eat no solid foods and drink only clear liquids. Your pelvic area may be shaved. It is important for you to let doctors and nurses know about any health issues, such as hypertension, heart disease, diabetes, or lung problems, as well as any drugs that you are presently taking.

Are blood transfusions needed during prostate operations?

Transfusions are sometimes needed during surgery for a radical prostatectomy, since as much as two pints of blood may be lost during surgery. Be sure to ask the doctor whether or not there is a possibility that you will need to have blood transfusions. Many men bank their own blood beforehand to eliminate any risk of receiving blood that has been contaminated with hepatitis, AIDS, or other transmissible diseases.

What is involved in banking blood?

Usually, a patient can donate a pint of blood every week or ten days for the month before surgery. Many doctors recommend that you take iron pills during this time to help assist your body in replacing your donated blood. Blood can be stored for about 45 days. You should have at least three days between the last donation and your surgery.

What kind of anesthesia is usually used for prostate cancer surgery?

Many doctors prefer epidural anesthesia, the narcotic often used for women during labor. The potent narcotic is given directly around the spinal cord, blocking pain but leaving you aware. Epidural anesthesia assures a total absence of pain, normal muscle function, and complete relaxation. Others use a spinal anesthetic that blocks all pain as well as the ability to feel and use the legs. However, spinal anesthesia is usually avoided if you have had back surgery or spinal cord injuries. General anesthesia can also be used to put you into a drug-induced sleep and to allow close control of vital functions especially if you have abnormally low blood pressure or certain types of heart problems. Muscle relaxants may be given during surgery to decrease the amount of general anesthetic needed.

Can I decide what kind of anesthesia I would like?

The decision on the kind of anesthesia is usually made by your anesthesiologist and surgeon. However, you should be sure to discuss any chronic health problems, medications, allergies, drug sensitivities, or preferences with your surgeon and anesthesiologist beforehand.

QUESTIONS TO ASK THE ANESTHESIOLOGIST

- What kind of medication will I be given before I am taken into the operating room?
- Who will be administering the medication and anesthesia?
- How will they be given to me?
- Are you an anesthesiologist or an anesthetist?
- Will my allergies be a problem?
- What kind of anesthetic are you going to give to me?
- What are the side effects?
- What are the risks?
- How long will the operation take?
- How long will it take before I regain consciousness?
- Will I go to a recovery room after the operation?
- What are the fees for your service?
- If you do not want to be fully unconscious during surgery, are elderly, or have lung problems, ask, Is general anesthesia absolutely necessary or is there another choice?

Who is responsible for anesthesia?

Anesthesia should be given either by an anesthesiologist or under the direction of an anesthesiologist. An anesthesiologist is a physician who specializes in anesthesia and is responsible for careful monitoring of bodily functions during the surgery. An anesthetist is usually a specially trained nurse who gives anesthesia under the direction of the doctor.

How long will the operation take?

Usually a radical prostatectomy will take between two and four hours, including the removal and examination of the lymph nodes of the pelvis. Tissue from the prostate and lymph nodes is sent to the pathologist during the operation so that it can be analyzed to see if the cancer has spread. This analysis, called a frozen section, is a rapid procedure that freezes the tissue quickly, giving the surgeon an almost immediate reading on the status of your cancer. Because the freezing process can distort the tissue and make it less accurate, the final result of the biopsy can take several days. This is called a permanent section biopsy and the results will be reported to you by your doctor.

How does the pathologist determine whether the tumor has spread beyond its margins?

When the tumor is removed and sent to the pathologist, it is painted with a substance similar to India ink. This colors the margins or outer edges of the prostate so that they can be examined and identified on the slides. If the cancer cells extend beyond the margins, then it is obvious that it has spread. If the cells are contained entirely within the margins, the tumor is said to be encapsulated, and usually no further treatment is recommended. If the margins are involved, additional postoperative radiation treatment will probably be recommended.

How long will it be before I know the results of the permanent section biopsy taken during the surgery?

It can be several days to a week before the final results of the biopsy are known. The tissue is put through a time-consuming multistage procedure that involves a series of solutions to remove water and fatty substances. It is then saturated with warm liquid paraffin. When it has cooled and hardened, the tissue in paraffin is cut into thin slices. The slices are placed on slides so that the tissue can be studied under the microscope.

Should I make arrangements for the doctor to talk with someone I designate as soon as the surgery is completed?

If you want someone to be able to talk to the doctor after your operation, to be involved with any decisions that might be necessary, or to be there when you come back to your room, make sure you tell your doctor who that person is and ask where the person should wait and how long the procedure will take. Some hospitals and surgicenters have a special waiting room while others will tell you to have family and friends wait in your room. Also, if you feel strongly that someone should **not** be given any information until you are alert, be sure to explain this to your doctor beforehand. These are all things you want to discuss before the operation.

Does the length of time I spend in the operating room indicate the seriousness of the operation?

It depends on the individual case. There are several situations that can make your time in the operating room longer but have no bearing on your own operation. For instance:

- You were taken from your room some time in advance of the actual operation.
- The anesthesiologist may make some additional preparations that last 30 minutes or even an hour.
- The surgeon takes longer than expected on the operation before yours, thus starting on your operation later than scheduled.
- You could spend more time than anticipated in the recovery room.

Those people who are waiting for you should understand that they should not judge the length or seriousness of the operation by the amount of time you spend in the operating room.

Will I need to go to a recovery room after my operation?

Yes. After the operation, you will be watched and checked by the medical team until you are stable enough to move. The recovery room has equipment for monitoring your heart action and a respirator for assisting you in breathing if you need it. You can get intravenous fluids and blood in the recovery room. Normally the recovery room is run by a physician anesthesiologist so that you can be monitored. Respiration therapists will probably help you cough and inflate your lungs. If you have had general anesthesia, you may spend several hours in the recovery room.

Will things seem hazy as I come out of general anesthesia?

Sometimes they do. Voices may seem very loud, or they may seem like they are coming from a long way off. People may seem to be moving differently from the way you think they should. You will probably feel groggy, your arms and legs may feel like lead, and you may feel cold. Vision, hearing, and sense of balance can all be affected by anesthesia, and it takes time for the effects to wear off. You will be half asleep, and until your vital signs are stable and there is no apparent problem, you will be kept in the recovery room.

How long does it take for the anesthesia to wear off after an operation?

Once the operation is finished, it can take anywhere from minutes to hours before it wears off, depending upon the kind of anesthesia you are given and the dose. Some people find that after general anesthesia they are light-headed for as long as a few days. Don't worry, it will pass and there will be no permanent effect from it.

Is it wise to have someone waiting in my room when I get out of the recovery room?

It is a good idea because someone who knows you may be able to spot problems more quickly. It will also be a comfort for you to know that someone is there even if you are drowsy or sleeping most of the time.

Is there a possibility of a blood clot following prostate surgery?

Blood clots are one of the most common causes of sudden death after surgery and can occur days or weeks after the operation. A pulmonary embolus is a large blood clot in a vein of the leg or pelvis that breaks loose. If it is large and reaches the heart, it can totally block blood flow and result in an almost instant drop of blood pressure.

What can be done to avoid the risk of blood clots?

During surgery, most doctors use special stockings that inflate and deflate to keep the blood flowing through the veins. After surgery, you will probably be given support stockings to wear. You will be helped to sit up and dangle your legs over the side of the bed. The day after surgery, you will be helped to get up and walk, and you will be encouraged to increase your walking daily. This will help speed your recovery and minimize the complications from surgery.

QUESTIONS TO ASK YOUR DOCTOR AFTER HAVING PROSTATE SURGERY

- How long will the catheter stay in place?
- Are bladder spasms to be expected?
- How long can I expect my urine to look cloudy?
- When will the stitches be removed?
- How long will the dribbling and feeling of urgency to urinate continue?
- How long can I expect to be incontinent?
- Are there exercises I can do to strengthen the muscles that control urination?
- When can I start driving a car; using stairs; lifting; walking; playing tennis, golf, or other active sports again?
- How long will it be before I am fully recuperated?

Will I be in pain following surgery?

You will have some postoperative pain that may require narcotics for relief. Many hospitals have patient-controlled analgesia machines so you can administer the pain-relieving medication as you need it so that pain and discomfort are minimized.

What is the purpose of the tube that's put down my throat?

Because there may be a slowdown in the normal intestinal contractions because organs were moved during the operation, a tube is sometimes placed through your nose and into your stomach and connected to a suction machine. Fluids that accumulate because of the lack of normal stomach and intestinal contractions are removed through the tube. It will probably be left in place for a few days, while you are in the hospital, until your body begins to work normally again and you begin to pass gas, which is a sign that things are back to normal. Once the tube is removed, you'll be able to eat normally.

Will I have a drain following surgery?

A drain, which runs from the site of the surgery through a small slit in the abdomen, allows blood, urine, or other fluids that would otherwise accumulate in the surgical area to be drained outside the body. Keeping the surgical areas free of these fluids promotes faster healing and lessens the possibility of infection.

Drains are usually removed after there is no more drainage, usually five to six days after surgery. Removal is not painful.

Is it common for testicles to be swollen after prostate surgery?

Because prostate surgery involves the nodes and ducts that normally drain the groin, thighs, and scrotum, these areas may be swollen for several weeks after surgery. As your body heals, this condition will subside.

Why is a catheter needed during and after surgery?

A catheter (also called a urinary tube or Foley catheter) is placed into the bladder at the time of surgery. It helps to drain the bladder during the period of healing and serves as a splint for healing around the area where the bladder neck is stitched to the stump of the urethra. Urine drains automatically through the catheter into a urine bag. You can keep discomfort to a minimum by keeping the end of your penis clean and softened with ointment. The catheter tube will be secured to your thigh with tape, and you may need to experiment to find the most comfortable angle for securing the catheter tube. Care must be taken to prevent accidental removal, so try to refrain from pulling on the catheter. Premature removal can interfere with recovery.

How long does the catheter remain in place?

Depending on your progress, the catheter usually remains in place for two to three weeks after radical prostatectomy. This means you will still have the catheter when you go home from the hospital. You will be taught how to care for it before you leave. You must make sure the catheter is well secured to the thigh and avoid traction and tension on it. Make sure that the tube between the penis and the bag is not obstructed by being crimped or pinched, especially at night. Keep the bag below the penis so that urine drains into the bag. If urine cannot flow from your bladder or flows back into the bladder, it can create bladder complications. After it is removed, there may be some dribbling and urgency to urinate for several weeks. For most individuals, this condition gradually improves as muscles heal and strengthen.

Do I have to wait until the catheter is removed before I can drive?

Most doctors suggest that you do not drive until your catheter has been removed. After the removal of the catheter (usually two to

three weeks), you should limit driving to short distances for another two weeks.

Are bladder spasms common after prostatectomy surgery?

Bladder spasms may occur after a prostatectomy. These spasms
have a rapid onset and usually subside in a few minutes. They can
be quite painful. Sometimes these spasms can be caused by the
obstruction of the catheter due to kinked tubing, mucous plugs,
or blood clots. Once the spasms start, you have little choice but
to relax as much as you can until the spasms subside. If the spasms
become too frequent for comfort, your doctor can prescribe an-
tispasmodic drugs.

Is it normal for my urine to be cloudy?

Your urine may be cloudy for several weeks after surgery. It will
clear up as the wound heals.

How long will convalescence take?

Convalescence time can vary, but most men are able to do all the
things they did prior to surgery after three or four months.

**What can be done if I find that, following surgery, I have difficulty
voiding?**

This should be reported to the doctor. It is a complication that
sometimes follows radical prostate surgery and usually means that
the bladder neck area that was stitched to the urethra has contracted, resulting in a restricted urinary stream. This can be re-
paired by the doctor either with a dilating instrument or surgically
through the urethra.

Is incontinence to be expected following a prostatectomy?

Many men are surprised to discover that the operation causes
them to lose their ability to control urine. They are embarrassed
to find that they must use incontinence pads to control dribbling.
Very often, incontinence will lessen as the healing continues. It
should continue to improve for up to six months or a year after
surgery. A small percentage of men who undergo radical prostatectomy will have total loss of bladder control. Many men report
that they must continue to wear pads to prevent leakage. Many
say they have intermittent dribbling caused by coughing or exer-
tion. Incontinence can sometimes be overcome through the

"As a doctor involved with a major cancer center, finding I had prostate cancer seemed at first like something I almost knew would happen to me," reports Dr. John. "My cancer was in the early stages, so after talking with both my surgical and radiology doctor friends, I decided to go with nerve-sparing prostate surgery.

"I must admit that being a patient gave me a totally different view of the practice of medicine. I tried to keep everything low key and not make a big deal of things. But when the dribbling didn't seem to stop a month after surgery and I was still wearing diapers after three months, I must admit I was very depressed. That problem continued for more than a year, but my muscle tone is better now after doing the Kegel exercises, and I've finally gotten rid of the pads. I've changed my life a lot, appreciating my family and my free time more than ever. I guess I was lucky my cancer was a Stage B where the nerve-sparing surgery was possible."

strengthening of muscles with simple exercise. (See Chapter 15 for more information on other methods of dealing with incontinence.)

How can I strengthen muscles to improve incontinence?

Corrective exercises (one type is referred to as Kegel exercises), designed to strengthen your perineal muscles, may be helpful.

- Empty your bladder. Try to relax yourself completely. Tense your muscles by pressing your buttocks together. Hold this position and count to ten. Relax and count to ten. Do this exercise for ten minutes each time, three times a day. At the beginning, you may not be able to hold the position for the count of ten or you may tire before you have completed the entire set. If so, stop exercising and go back to it later.
- When starting to void, shut off the stream for a few seconds, then start voiding again. Do this exercise each time you urinate to improve urinary control.
- Remember to urinate as soon as you feel the need. Do not wait.

- It may take several weeks or months of daily exercise before you notice a difference.

When can I resume sexual activities after a prostatectomy?

If you had nerve-sparing surgery, it may take six months to a year or two before you are able to achieve an erection, but you can usually resume sexual activity within six weeks following surgery when the operative site is healed.

Following a prostatectomy, is radiation sometimes recommended?

It depends on what has been found during surgery and whether your PSA level returns to normal. In some cases, for example, when the surgery shows that the cancer has spread beyond the prostate capsule or into the seminal vesicles or the PSA level remains elevated three weeks after surgery, postoperative radiation may be necessary.

What is lymphedema?

Lymphedema is an accumulation of lymph fluid that may cause swelling in the legs following the removal of lymph nodes (lymphadenectomy). Not being able to drain, the lymph fluid remains in the soft tissue, where infections can develop. People who have had lymph node dissection are at greatest risk. Lymphedema is most commonly seen in women who have had axillary nodes removed during breast cancer surgery. However, lymphedema may also occur in men who have had surgery or radiation therapy for prostate cancer. Curiously enough, not everyone who has lymph node surgery has lymphedema. Lymphedema, however, can occur soon after surgery or even as many as 15 years after surgery.

Does lymphedema mean my cancer has spread?

Many people fear that lymphedema means that the cancer has spread or returned. Another fear is that the swollen, nonfunctional limb may be permanently disfigured. It is important to discuss your fears with the health care professionals in your life, so that they can help you to learn the necessary measures you need to take to keep lymphedema under control. Positioning, massage, exercise, special garments, and pumps are all used in treating lymphedema.

How can you tell if you have lymphedema?

About half of patients who have lymphedema report a feeling of heaviness or fullness in the affected area. A slight indentation may be visible when the skin on the limb is pressed. Depending on how extensive the problem is, a deep fingerprint may take any-where from 5 to 30 seconds to disappear. At the extreme, the limb may swell to one and a half to two times its normal size. You should always be aware of any signs of infection in the involved area—redness, pain, heat, chills, swelling, or fever. Though rare, infections can move quickly and become serious very rapidly.

How important is it to get immediate care?

Immediate care is essential. Untreated, the condition can result in a permanently swollen leg. Awareness of the possibility of lym-phedema and the need for immediate medical attention may help to keep the problem from becoming chronic. Obesity; immobility; poor nutrition; prior radiation or surgery; and concurrent medi-cal problems, such as diabetes, hypertension, kidney disease, cardiac disease, and phlebitis, can all be contributing factors to the onset of lymphedema. Those who have any of those problems should be extremely aware of the symptoms and the need for lifelong adherence to prevention and control of lymphedema.

Where can I get information about lymphedema?

The National Lymphedema Network provides printed informa-tion and other assistance to those who develop lymphedema as a result of lymph node surgery or radiation therapy. The address is 2211 Post Street, Suite 404, San Francisco, CA 94115. The tele-phone number is 1-800-541-3259. See Chapter 16 for more re-source information.

chapter 9

What Happens If I Have External Radiation?

> Radiation has been used for prostate cancer treatment since the 1950s. External-beam radiation, today's most commonly used radiation treatment, involves directing a beam of radiation at the prostate gland to destroy the tumor. This treatment usually consists of a series of 30 to 40 daily treatments, requiring a visit to a radiation facility five days a week for six to eight weeks. Be sure to check the type of radiation equipment that will be used in your treatment. The number of radiation oncology facilities that have access to the most advanced technology is limited at this time. Talk to your doctor about the kind of equipment that will be used for your treatment.

There is still controversy among physicians about the circumstances under which radiation is most effective for treating prostate cancer. However, according to some authorities, it appears that when similarly staged patients are treated with surgery or radiation and carefully compared at the end of 10 years, there is little difference in the outcome. In addition, again according to limited studies, there is little basis for the belief that younger patients should be treated with surgery because they will live longer, or the patient sacrifices a survival advantage when he selects radiation treatment.

At 10 years, however, there is some evidence that increasing PSA levels and local recurrences become more common in men who have had radiation treatment than in those who have had surgery. What is still not resolved is whether these differences are due to the fact that men who had prostate surgery were less advanced at the start than those who had external radiation treatment.

Like other treatments for prostate cancer, external radiation has some serious aftereffects. In a group of 100 men who have had prostate radiation, it has been shown that the following side effects may be expected:

Impotence	40
Some long-term incontinence	6
Severe incontinence	7
Difficult urination	5
Rectal problems	11
Severe rectal problems	2

What are the advantages and disadvantages of radiation treatment?

Radiation is ideal for the man who cannot or does not wish to have his prostate removed or whose health makes surgery a higher risk. It avoids many of the risks of surgery and anesthesia, such as surgical bleeding, hospitalization, pain, or heart attacks, strokes, or blood clots. There is a risk of developing some degree of bladder or rectal irritation. Some of the side effects, such as bloody urine or impotence, can appear months or years after treatment.

What kind of doctor should I go to for radiation treatments?

Radiation is a very specialized field, requiring treatment from a team especially trained in therapeutic radiology. The radiation oncologist, sometimes called a therapeutic radiologist, heads the team and plans the treatment. The radiation oncologist will decide what specific treatments should be used, supervise its administration, and evaluate you at intervals during the course of the treatment to see whether it is working.

Who are the other members of the radiation team?

This will vary from place to place, but there are usually several other people who work with the radiation oncologist. The radiation physicist and the dosimetrist help in calculating the dose, planning the exact treatment field, creating special blocks or shields, and devising other treatment set-up aids. They use a computer to plan the treatment and to calculate the distribution of the radiation dose. The radiation therapist or technologist is the person who is responsible for following the plan, getting you ready for treatment, and giving your daily treatment. The radiation therapy nurse is an oncology nurse with specialized training in your care during radiation and in helping to manage any side effects. A dietitian, a physical therapist, a social worker, or other health care professionals may also be part of the team's services.

Will I have a choice as to where I have my radiation treatments?

It is a good idea for you to have a frank discussion with your doctor about why a specific radiation oncologist or radiotherapy department is being recommended. You may want to explore whether it would be advantageous for you to use a larger medical center versus a small hospital or private office closer to home. A large radiation center will have several types of equipment and beams to use for treatment, whereas a smaller general hospital or private office may be limited to less sophisticated equipment. You must weigh for yourself the advantages of convenience versus the technology and expertise a larger medical center may have to offer. Of course, your type of health insurance may put some limitations on where you can receive your treatment. Radiation treatment is a science in which many advances have been made in both technology and application. The radiation team and the equipment will be playing an important part in your treatment. **Be sure to check to see if there is a center near you that is** using computers to achieve three-dimensional planning and treatment.

QUESTIONS TO ASK YOUR RADIATION ONCOLOGIST BEFORE HAVING RADIATION TREATMENTS

- Exactly what type of radiation treatment will I be getting?
- Will it be done with a high-energy linear accelerator?
- Is three-dimensional conformal radiation available anywhere in the area?
- Are you planning to do a lymph node dissection? If yes, why?
- Do you advise hormone treatment to reduce the cancer before radiation?
- Who will be responsible for coordinating my radiation treatment? For giving my treatment?
- If I have questions about my radiation treatment, whom should I ask?
- Can I continue to work during these treatments?
- Is there a more convenient place where my treatments can be given?
- How long will it take for each treatment? For the whole series?
- Will I be able to drive myself to my treatments?
- What side effects can I expect?
- What should I do if these side effects occur?
- What side effects should I report to the radiation oncologist?
- How much will it cost? Is it covered by insurance?
- What are the risks of my becoming incontinent or impotent?
- What other side effects does radiation cause?
- Are there any alternatives to external-beam radiation treatment I should consider?
- When will you be checking my PSA again? How rapidly should I expect it to drop?
- If a biopsy is suggested earlier than 18 months after radia-

tion treatment, ask, "What information do you expect to get from a biopsy at this time?"

What is involved with external-beam radiation therapy?

You will go to a hospital or radiation facility for a period of time— usually five days a week for six to eight weeks. Rays are aimed at the tumor and the area around it. The treatment itself takes only a few minutes. Toward the end of treatment, an extra "boost" of radiation is often given to a smaller area of the pelvis where most of the tumor is located.

What is the most effective kind of radiation equipment?

An important factor to check out if you are planning to have external radiation is the type of machinery that will be used in your radiation treatment. A high-energy linear accelerator is the most effective for treating the pelvic area. Many radiation oncologists feel that low-energy photons or cobalt-60 units can cause a higher incidence of complications. A total of 6,000 to 7,200 rads is usually given over the entire treatment period.

What is three-dimensional conformal radiation?

Three-dimensional conformal radiation is a new technology, presently undergoing clinical trials. It allows radiation doses to be increased significantly because its accuracy makes it possible to pinpoint prostate tumors so that even adjacent normal tissue is spared from radiation. This computer-based system creates a very accurate picture of the prostate, enabling radiation oncologists to fashion multiple beams that are shaped exactly to the contour of the prostate gland. The technique makes it safer to deliver a maximum dose of high-energy x-rays directly to the tumor.

Are there some men who are at higher risk for complications after radiation treatments for their prostate cancers?

Men who are at increased risk for major complications after treatment include those who have had a number of TURPs (transurethral resections of the prostate) in their history; those with bladder infections or kidney stones; those who have autoimmune diseases such as lupus, ulcerative colitis, or enteritis; and those who have had multiple prior abdominal surgeries.

Are younger men with prostate cancer better off having prostate surgery rather than radiation?

This is a question that will continue to be debated among physicians. The very respected medical book *Cancer: Principles & Practice of Oncology*, fourth edition, edited by Drs. Vincent T. DeVita, Jr., Samuel Hellman, and Steven A. Rosenberg, states in its chapter on prostate cancer: "There is no basis in fact for the frequently made statements that younger patients should be treated with surgery because they will live longer, that radiation shows late failure, and that the patient sacrifices a survival advantage when he selects radiation treatment." So, for younger men, as for all other men with prostate cancer, the important thing to remember is that you need to study the pros and cons of each treatment and how they will affect your life. You need to understand your own case before making a decision on treatment.

Is hormone treatment sometimes prescribed before radiation is given?

Some doctors recommend that hormonal therapy be given before or during radiation to debulk, or reduce the size of, the tumor and make it more manageable for treatment. Hormonal treatment in addition to radiation is presently in clinical trials.

Does radiation treatment get rid of the cancer permanently?

As with surgery, about half of the men who have radiation may still have positive biopsy results for cancer two to three years after treatment. Some studies seem to imply that biopsies taken within 18 to 24 months after radiation treatment may be unreliable because this slow-growing tumor also regresses slowly.

Is it wise for me to consider having a laparoscopic lymphadenectomy before having radiation to determine whether the cancer has spread?

The reason for doing a lymphadenectomy is to help in the medical management and decisions involved with treating the cancer. It has no therapeutic or curative value. Lymphadenectomy is considered by many doctors to be a less than perfect procedure. If positive nodes are found and a different treatment is decided upon, then it may be worthwhile. But if the treatment will remain the same whether the nodes are found to be negative or positive, you may well decide you do not want to submit to the procedure. One of the rare but possible side effects that can be troublesome when a lymphadenectomy is followed by radiation is the possibility of leg and genital lymphedema (swelling). Lymphedema is caused by impaired lymphatic drainage, sometimes appearing years after treatment. When chronic lymphedema develops, it is a lifelong condition that requires constant monitoring and therapy. (See Chapter 8 for additional information on lymphedema.)

What is a laparoscopic lymphadenectomy?

This procedure, which is done to determine if the cancer has already spread to the lymph nodes, uses four puncture wounds of about one-half inch each rather than a single vertical incision. It is performed *inside* the intestinal or abdominal cavity. This procedure has an increased risk of bowel obstruction because of adhesions or injury. Though it sounds simple, the procedure takes two to four hours to perform, but you will usually be able to go home the next day. If your doctor suggests a laparoscopic lymphadenectomy, be sure to ask why it is being done and how the information will change or modify your planned treatment. (The standard lymphadenectomy is performed through a six-inch vertical lower abdominal incision outside the abdominal cavity without exposing the abdominal cavity to surgical trauma.)

Is radiation used for treating prostate cancer that has already been treated with surgery?

Radiation is used following a prostatectomy in many cases where it is found that there are positive nodes or positive surgical margins. (See Chapter 3 for information on surgical margins.) It is usually given soon after recovery from surgery. A lower radiation dose can be used if given soon after surgery rather than waiting until there are signs of problems.

Is radiation effective for treatment of prostate cancer that has spread to the lymph nodes?

Just as surgical removal of the prostate does not remove cancer that has spread to the lymph nodes, radiation rarely cures prostate

Chris had been a hard-working construction worker who had just recently retired and was planning to move to Florida when he discovered he had prostate cancer. A practical kind of guy, he looked at his options, and because he was given a choice of either an operation or radiation, he decided to go with the radiation. He admits that he didn't do a lot of reading or checking out of treatments. He just went with what his doctor told him. He says he was really scared when he first heard the diagnosis. However, it has now been five years since he finished radiation treatments, and although he reports that he did have some complications at the time, that's all in the past. He says that he has had some problems with erections, but he feels that this is probably due to age.

Sixty-eight-year-old Charlie, on the other hand, was handed a prostate cancer diagnosis two years ago when his PSA came back a 5. The first doctor he went to told him to have a prostatectomy immediately and had him booked for an operation the next week. Being a methodical sort, he decided to check out a radiation oncologist at a nearby cancer center. After the doctor looked at his records and talked with him at length about his options, Charlie decided he liked this doctor's approach and that radiation better suited his lifestyle. And the odds against impotence and incontinence were better, too. Even though he's had some diarrhea problems, Charlie says he's very happy with his decision. He is active in a local support group, where he feels he can help other men who are faced with making tough decisions.

cancer that has already spread. However, it is sometimes used to treat symptoms.

If I have recently had a TURP procedure, when can I start radiation?

For those who have had a prior TURP, radiation is usually delayed for four to six weeks after the operation to allow for complete healing.

Will radiation effect my blood counts?

Sometimes it may. The radiation oncologist may find you have low white blood cell counts or low levels of platelets, which can affect your body's ability to fight infection and prevent bleeding. If your blood tests show these problems, you may have to go off treatment for a week or so to allow your blood counts to come back up.

What steps will the radiation oncologist take in planning my external radiation treatments?

The radiation oncologist will thoroughly examine you and study your x-rays, computerized tomographic scans, pathology slides, hospital records, and any other pertinent information about your case. Then the radiation oncologist will discuss the recommendations on the type and duration of radiation treatment. The next step probably will be a treatment planning session.

Will I have my first treatment at my first appointment with the radiation oncologist?

Probably not, although it depends on how complex your case is. It is highly unlikely that you will have your first treatment during your first appointment, because your treatment plan needs to be set up. Treatment plans are different for each patient, so it may take more than one visit before your treatment actually begins.

How is the radiation dose decided upon?

The dose varies with the size of the tumor, the extent of the tumor, the tumor type and grade, and its response to radiation. Computers are used to determine the treatment volume and the distribution of the dose within that volume. Several plans may be generated from which the radiation oncologist will select the one that provides the desired distribution of the dose.

How will I be shielded from unnecessary radiation?

There are many safeguards to protect you from unnecessary radiation to the parts of your body that do not need treatment. All the machines are designed so that the large amounts of radiation are given only to a specific area. The treatment field is usually lit with a light that outlines the surface through which the radiation will pass. A series of safeguards in the machine limits the radiation to this lighted area of your body. Shields, usually made out of lead blocks, are used to protect small areas of your body not needing treatment. Custom-made casts of plaster or plastic are also used.

How are the casts made?

You will be put in the position you will assume during treatment. The cast is made right on your body, using a material such as plaster, plastic, or Styrofoam. Small windows are cut into the mold to allow the beam to be directed to the precise area to be treated. The radiation oncologist can use the mold on you over and over again to be sure the beam is always directed to the proper area.

How will the spot where the radiation is to be given be marked?

Once the location has been decided, the radiation oncologist or the radiation therapist will draw marks on your skin to outline the area to receive treatment. Marking pens, indelible ink, or silver nitrate may be used. You will be asked not to wash away these markings. After your first week of treatment, you may have permanent markings put on your skin. Usually, small pinpoint tattoos placed at the corners of the treatment field are used.

How is the permanent tattoo done?

It is a very simple process, which is a substitute for the ink markings used for your early treatments. A drop of India ink is placed on your skin, and with a needle, a tiny permanent dot is made on the skin itself.

Is the treatment plan ever changed?

Your original radiation treatment plan may be added to, subtracted from, or changed as the radiation oncologist feels is appropriate. There are a number of reasons for making changes as the treatment progresses. Do not be alarmed if the plan is changed. It does not mean that the disease is getting worse or that the disease has progressed.

Why is the radiation treatment sometimes given from different angles?

One way of giving the maximum amount of radiation to the tumor and the minimum amount to normal tissue is by aiming radiation beams at the tumor from two or more directions. The patient or the machine is rotated. The patient and the machine are placed so that the beams focus where the tumor is located. The tumor thus gets a high enough dose of radiation to be destroyed but normal surrounding tissues escape with minimum radiation effects because the beams take different pathways to reach the tumor.

Why is the radiation given over a period of time instead of all at once?

The radiation must be strong enough to kill the tumor and still allow the normal tissues to heal. The radiation oncologist determines the total radiation dose necessary and divides it into the number of single-treatment doses that will add up to this total dose by the time of the last treatment. This process, dividing the doses of radiation, is known as fractionation. Fractionation is a very important part of planning and delivering radiation because it affects both the tumor and the normal tissues.

Will my normal cells be affected by radiation?

All cells are affected by the radiation, whether they are normal or malignant. The normal tissues have a greater capacity to recover from the damage induced by the radiation than do the cancer cells. The radiation oncologist plans the treatment so that normal tissues are irradiated as little as possible.

What happens to the PSA after radiation treatment?

Don't be upset if your PSA level does not immediately drop to zero. The PSA level should drop below 1.0 over a period of several months. Some doctors think that the slower the PSA drops, the more successful the treatment.

Is it wise to have a biopsy after radiation to see if the treatment was effective?

As with the PSA test, biopsies done shortly after radiation are believed to be less accurate than those done between 18 and 24 months after treatment. It is generally believed that the results of biopsies done within the first 18 months after external radiation treatment may be unreliable and should be avoided.

Will I be able to drive myself to my treatments?

Many men are able to drive themselves to their treatments. As treatment progresses, however, some prefer to have their family and friends drive them. It depends on how well you feel in general and the side effects you are having. You need to discuss these issues with your nurse and radiation oncologist. If you need help with transportation, discuss it with the nurse at the radiation facility. Many times you can get rides through services in your own community, such as the American Cancer Society, community groups, senior citizen transportation services, or civic organizations.

Will I be alone in the room during treatment?

The radiation therapist will leave the room and will control the machine from the control room. You will be watched on a television screen. The machine, which is very large, will make a steady buzzing noise while the beam is on. Some treatment machines rotate around you, making a noise as they move. If you are concerned about what will happen in the treatment room, make sure you discuss it with the radiation therapist or the radiation oncology nurse before you begin your treatments.

Why can't the radiation therapist stay in the room with me while I am having my radiation treatment?

The machine, although it pinpoints the beam at a specific part of the body, does scatter some of the radiation. Although the amount of radiation outside the beam is tiny during any one radiation treatment session, over months and years, it could add up to a dangerous amount for the treatment personnel. It is important for the staff who are working with radiation all day long not to be exposed to these scattered beams. All personnel who are working with radiation must be carefully monitored with badges that measure their accumulated doses so that they will be able to tell if they have any unusual radiation exposures.

How long do the treatments take?

The actual treatment lasts from one to five minutes. You are usually in the treatment room for five to fifteen minutes for each treatment. The most usual schedule is to have a treatment each day for five days, with weekends off. Usually, you do not have treatments on holidays.

What is the actual treatment like?

Most people say that they feel nothing while the treatment is being given. A few say that they feel warmth or a mild tingling sensation. You will feel no pain or discomfort, and it will be unusual if you have any kind of sensation. If by any chance you do feel ill or very uncomfortable during the treatment, tell the radiation therapist. The machine can be stopped at any time. You need to remain very still during treatment, but you can breathe normally. Try to relax. Some people bring their headsets and soothing music into the treatment room with them. You may feel cold in the treatment room, because the temperature is kept cool for the proper operation of the machine.

Will the radiation I am getting make me radioactive?

No. External-beam radiation does not cause your body to become radioactive. There is no need to avoid being with other people because of your treatment. You can hug, kiss, and have sexual relations with others.

Will I have tests each time I go for my radiation treatments?

There may be some tests during the course of the treatment but not each time. It will depend on your treatment plan. Usually, tests such as blood counts are taken so that the radiation oncologist knows whether the radiation is doing damage to other parts of your body. Sometimes x-rays and other tests are needed to determine if the radiation oncologist should change the treatment plan.

Are there some general dos and don'ts for people getting radiation treatment?

Yes, there are some general guidelines. While you are having your radiation treatment, you need to take a few extra precautions to protect your overall good health and help the treatment succeed.

- Be sure to get plenty of rest. Sleep as often as you feel the need. Your body will use a lot of extra energy over the course of the treatment.
- Eating well is important. Try to maintain a diet that will prevent weight loss.

- Do not remove the ink marks from your skin. Do not draw over the faded lines at home. Some centers use small permanent tattoo marks.
- Tell the radiation oncologist about any medicine you are taking before you start treatment. If you need to take medicine, even aspirin, let your radiation oncologist know before you start. You also need to tell the radiation oncologist if your medicines are changed during your treatment. If you are taking medication for a chronic disease such as diabetes, and you are eating less while you are having treatment, your insulin dose may need to be changed.

What kinds of side effects can be expected from external radiation therapy?

Many men who have radiation therapy are able to continue their normal routines, although during the last weeks of therapy, many complain of feeling very tired. But most men find that about three months after treatment they are back to normal. Mild diarrhea is commonly reported as are rectal soreness, skin reactions, abdominal cramping, hemorrhoids, and cystitis. Many of the complications are temporary and usually clear up after a few weeks.

Other possible aftereffects include:

- Some temporary pain upon ejaculation and a permanent decrease in semen volume.
- Impotence (usually occurs in 40 percent of men who have radiation treatment for prostate cancer).
- Rectal bleeding (common due to ulceration of the rectal wall, where the radiation dosage is concentrated). This can usually be treated with enemas containing steroids or by laser.
- In rare cases, it may be necessary to have a temporary colostomy to allow time for healing.
- Incontinence and swelling of the legs and genital area (lymphedema) are less frequent side effects.

Will I lose my hair as a result of radiation?

The hair on your head will not fall out because of radiation, but there may be changes in the hair on your lower abdomen or pubic area. Usually the hair in those areas will thin out because of the radiation.

What can I do if I feel tired?

The feeling of tiredness should gradually begin to wear off within a few weeks after your treatment ends. The following should help:

- Eat when you feel tired. Sometimes a small amount of food will give you the extra energy you need.
- Rest when you feel tired. Some people get tired more quickly and need more rest during this time. Try to get more sleep at night. Rest during the day if you can. Don't feel you must keep up your normal schedule of activities if you feel tired. Use your leisure time in restful ways.
- Reduce your activities. You may wish to take some time off from work or work a reduced schedule for a while.
- Don't be afraid to ask family, friends, and neighbors for help.

Why would I have rectal soreness as the result of radiation?

Rectal soreness (referred to as proctitis) can be the result of radiation damage to the intestinal tract. A low-residue diet often will help to allow healing. Some doctors suggest the use of steroid enemas or suppositories to help alleviate symptoms. Antidiarrhea medication is sometimes prescribed.

What can be done about cystitis caused by radiation?

Cystitis, the inflammation of the bladder that causes pain upon urination, usually occurs during the first few weeks of therapy. You should try to drink at least 2 quarts of fluid each day. The doctor may also prescribe antispasmodics and analgesics to help alleviate some of the symptoms.

What can be done if I experience diarrhea?

Diarrhea can be one of the side effects. It can cause you to lose fluids and become dehydrated. Be sure to drink plenty of clear liquids (apple juice, clear broth, water, ginger ale) and eat foods that are high in potassium (bananas, oranges, potatoes). A diet that is low in roughage (raw vegetables, bran, beans, fresh fruit) and high in low-fiber foods (yogurt, mashed potatoes, chicken, turkey, white rice, and noodles) is best. Be sure to discuss the problem with your doctor if the diarrhea persists. You can get more information about diet and radiation by calling the Cancer Information Service, 1-800-4-CANCER, and asking for the booklet "Eating Hints."

What happens when there is damage to the bladder due to radiation?

Bladder damage can result from radiation treatment, causing urinary frequency that may make it necessary for you to go to the bathroom often, day and night. Bleeding from the bladder is another possible side effect. If bleeding occurs, call your doctor.

What are the side effects of external radiation therapy?

There is a chance with external-beam radiation that serious, permanent injury to the bowel and bladder may result. For this reason, it is essential that your radiation treatment be done by a qualified radiation oncologist who understands sophisticated radiation techniques, such as the use of linear accelerators and careful simulation and treatment planning.

Will I become incontinent as a result of external radiation therapy?

Although you may have some difficulty in urination, including pain and increased frequency, incontinence is not usually a major side effect of external radiation. Acute, temporary reactions may occur, but chronic problems or late reactions are unusual. (See Chapter 15 for more information on dealing with incontinence.)

Will I become impotent after radiation treatment?

Radiation can affect erections by damaging the arteries that carry blood to the penis. As the irradiated area heals, internal tissues may become scarred. The walls of the arteries may lose their elasticity so that they can no longer expand enough to let blood speed in and create a firm erection. So it is possible that although potency is preserved at the start, it may diminish over time. (See Chapter 15 for more information on sexual side effects.)

How do I keep my skin from becoming irritated?

Because the skin in the treated area is more sensitive, you need to take steps to try not to irritate it. Don't scrub it with a washcloth or a brush. Don't use soaps, creams, lotions, or powders on it without first checking with the nurse or radiation therapist. Don't apply anything hot or cold to it. Don't scratch or rub the skin in that area. Do not use adhesive tape because your skin is sensitive and may peel off with the tape. Wear loose-fitting clothes. If you do see an irritation or if your skin looks like it is going to blister or crack, be sure you report it to your radiation oncologist.

What do I do if I get skin reactions due to radiation?

Skin reactions in prostate cancer are quite rare, but may occur several weeks after radiation is begun. The irradiated area should be kept clean and dry. The skin should not be exposed to extreme heat or cold. Commercial skin creams or lotions should be avoided because some contain metal bases, which can cause further burning. Some water-based lotions, such as Aquaphor, may be used with approval of the radiation oncologist.

Will my skin get darker or redder?

It depends on the condition and color of your skin, the kind of radiation, your age and physical condition, and medications you might be taking. Most people do not see any changes during the first two weeks of treatment. Some people get little reaction at all. Others find their skin looks light pink or red, sunburned, or tanned. Sometimes it turns a bit rough and might even peel slightly. You may find that your skin is not as flexible or as movable as before. Tell your radiation oncologist or nurse when you first note reddening of your skin. If you are taking any medicines, make sure you tell the radiation oncologist and nurse what they are, so that they decide whether they need to monitor your skin more closely during treatment.

May I go swimming while I am having my radiation treatments?

You probably can as long as it does not cause your skin to dry out. You need to rinse your skin well with fresh water if you have been swimming in salt water or in a pool with chlorine in it. Be sure to avoid direct sun on the treated area.

Can I continue my usual activities during treatment?

Continue doing as much as you can without feeling tired and strained. Many people find they can continue to work during the treatment period. This is a time to listen to your body and to take good care of yourself. In addition, your radiation oncologist may suggest that you limit some activities, such as sports.

Do Medicare and Medicaid pay for radiation treatments?

Both Medicare and Medicaid cover the major portion of the cost of treatment. For Medicare, if the radiation oncologist is a participating physician (one who has agreed to accept the charges established by Medicare), the physician will be paid 80 percent of the recognized charge. You will pay the other 20 percent. If you have a Medigap insurance policy, it will usually cover the 20 percent copayment. Be sure you are not confused by the billing balance that some radiation oncologists who are not participating physicians add to your copayment bill. For instance, if Medicare pays $100 as the reasonable charge, a nonparticipating radiation oncologist may charge $120 for the procedure. Medicare would pay the patient or physician $80. If you pay the $20 copayment, $20 will remain as the billing balance. You should be aware that some states have legislated against the practice of balance billing.

chapter 10

What Happens If I Have Radiation Seeding?

Radiation seeding, sometimes called internal radiation, interstitial implantation, or brachytherapy, selectively places radioactive particles or seeds into the prostate. A number of years ago, the only way to do this was with abdominal surgery. Some trials at that time showed that because there was no way for the physician to pinpoint distribution of the implants, this method did not have satisfactory long-term results. The use of ultrasound now makes it possible for the seeds to be distributed evenly into the cancerous prostate in a larger dose without an abdominal incision. Stronger doses of radiation may be given in a more direct manner than when delivered externally. The effectiveness of this type of radiation seeding is presently being tested in clinical trials.

Radiation seeding was used extensively in the 1970s with abdominal surgery and freehand implantation of gold or iodine seeds. Because there was no way to check where the seeds were placed, studies showed that this method was not as successful as external radiation over the long term and was discontinued. New techniques—including using ultrasound for more precise seed placement and faster-acting iridium or palladium seeds—have made it possible to reevaluate this treatment. Studies are in progress to test various radioactive sources with ultrasound imaging. Because the new methods have been in use five years or less, the long-term results of these implant treatments are not yet available. However, it is felt that because of the stronger doses of radiation and the direct delivery, this method may, in time, prove to be the best answer to treating prostate cancer.

Like prostate surgery and external-beam radiation, internal radiation seeding has some serious aftereffects. Although not as many studies have been carried out with this treatment, there is some information about side effects. In a group of 100 men who have had internal seeding, it has been shown that the following side effects may be expected:

Impotence	25
Incontinence	0–2
With TURP	15
Serious rectal problems	20

Who is the best candidate for radiation seeding?

Radiation seeding implants are most appropriate in men with small or well- or moderately differentiated cancers and men in whom surgery is considered a high risk for other reasons.

What kind of doctor does radiation seeding?

Since this treatment is fairly new, you need to seek out a radiation oncologist who has had experience in this technique. Radiation seeding theoretically should be more effective than external radiation because the seeds deliver as much as two and a half times the dose to the prostate without affecting nearby organs. However, if not placed properly, they can injure the urethra, bladder, or rectum. Therefore, the expertise of the radiation oncologist is of primary importance.

How is radiation seeding done?

Radiation seeding is usually done with the help of ultrasound and computer. The doctor implants radioactive material directly into

Sam was found to have an irregular lump on one side of his prostate five years ago when he was 53. After researching all the options, he decided to go with a clinical trial of radiation seeds. Weighing heavily in his decision was the fact that this treatment seemed to be the best way to preserve his sex life.

"I had too many friends who told me horror stories about their prostate operations and the problems they had with diapers and no erections. To me this seemed like the perfect answer to my problem. My PSA is low, and my doctor says everything checks out fine. As far as sexual activity goes, I did have some problems with erections at first, and though my erections aren't as strong as they once were, I still get a great deal of pleasure out of sex. When I hear what's happened to other guys who've had some of the other treatments, I consider myself very lucky."

the tumor with long needles passed through the perineum. Radioactive iodine, iridium, and palladium are most commonly used. The procedure and results are presently under clinical evaluation. Another experimental seed implantation technique, called high-dose-rate radiation, attaches seeds to a wire inserted into the patient's prostate through a number of hollow tubes, one after the other. Doctors feel that the use of ultrasound imaging techniques for guiding implantation directly to the cancer is a big step forward in perfecting this technique.

QUESTIONS TO ASK YOUR RADIATION ONCOLOGIST BEFORE HAVING RADIATION SEEDING

- Do you think internal radiation seeding will work for me?
- How many of these procedures have you done? What are the results?
- What kind of radioactive material will you be using?
- How will the radioactive material be put in my body?
- Are you planning a lymph node dissection? How will it be done? Why is it being done? Is it necessary?
- Will I need anesthesia? Will it be local or general?

- How long will I need to be in the hospital for this procedure?
- Will I have to stay in bed during this time?
- Will I be able to have visitors? Will there be any restrictions on the visitors?
- Will the implant be permanent?
- Will I be radioactive while the implant is inside me? For how long?
- What side effects should I expect?
- When will it be safe to have intercourse?
- When will I be able to get back to my normal routine?
- How much will it cost?
- Will my health insurance cover the treatment?

Is hormonal treatment ever used before seed implantation?

The use of hormonal therapy for a period of up to six months prior to treatment can help to decrease the tumor volume and size of the prostate and may make the radiation seeding treatment more effective.

How is radiation seeding planned?

Using ultrasound scans, your physician will create a map of your prostate. This will be used to calculate the exact number of seeds for complete coverage and accurate placement. Usually 40 to 100 seeds are implanted in the prostate gland. A treatment planning computer constructs the implant model to optimize radiation distribution.

What does the treatment involve?

After spinal or general anesthesia, an ultrasound probe is positioned in the rectum to allow for proper needle alignment. A template guidance device, which is attached to the ultrasound probe, has holes that correspond to the grid on the ultrasound computer screen. Implant needles are put through the appropriate template holes. These needles may be preloaded with the seeds or may attach to an applicator that dispenses the radioactive seeds through the needle and into the prostate. Each needle is guided through the template, then through the perineum (the area between the rectum and scrotum) to its predetermined position. The ultrasound unit's screen allows the physician to see the needle's exact position in the prostate. A predetermined number of seeds are then implanted. When all seeds have been inserted, the ultrasound image is again reviewed to verify seed placement.

How long does this procedure take to complete?

The actual procedure takes about an hour to complete. Often it is done as an outpatient or overnight procedure under spinal or general anesthesia. You will be in the recovery room until the effects of the anesthesia have disappeared. An antibiotic will usually be prescribed.

What are the possible complications of radiation seeding?

There may be bruising and swelling between the legs, which disappears in a few days. Urinary discomfort—a sense of urgency, burning during urination, slight bleeding, or blood in the urine—is to be expected but will diminish as the seeds lose their radioactivity usually within three months. Rectal irritation and occasional rectal bleeding may occur but should subside in less than three months.

Can I have radiation seeding if I previously had a TURP?

If you previously had a TURP (transurethral resection of the prostate), the changes in your prostate gland make it difficult to uniformly distribute seeds, so radiation seeding is usually not recommended.

Does the PSA usually fall after this treatment?

PSA values usually fall back to the normal range within three to six months after implantation.

Is radiation seeding sometimes combined with external radiation?

Sometimes when the cancer is locally advanced, external radiation will be used before or following the implant procedure.

Is lymph node dissection (lymphadenectomy) done before radiation seeding?

Sometimes lymph node dissection is done to determine if the cancer has spread to the lymph nodes. The dissection is usually not done if the cancer is low grade and the PSA level is low.

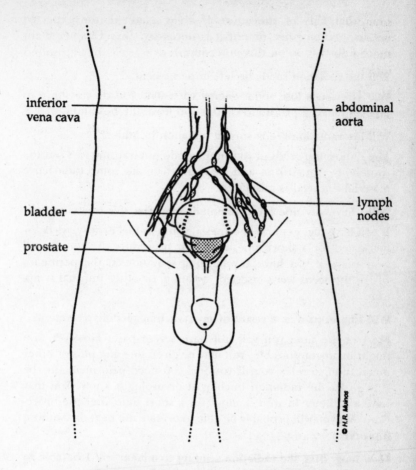

**Lymph node dissection removes some of
lymph nodes that drain lymphatic fluid from prostate.**

Generally, the laparoscopic method of lymph node dissection is
used instead of an abdominal lymph node operation. Some physicians feel that laparoscopic lymphadenectomy is not as accurate
as an abdominally performed lymph node dissection. It is possible
to do the laparoscopic lymph node dissection at the same time as
the seeding, but the two procedures are most often done separately. Before agreeing to lymph node dissection, be sure to ques-

tion what type of procedure is being planned, the expected results, and whether or not it is necessary. (See Chapter 8 for more information on this procedure.)

Will the radiation seeds be left in permanently?

Yes. The seeds lose some energy each day. You do not have to take any special precautions after you leave the hospital.

Will the radiation seeds spread radiation to others?

The radioactive seeds in your implant do not transmit rays outside your body. Your urine and stool may contain some radioactive material if a seed is misplaced.

Will I have any side effects immediately after this treatment?

If you have had general anesthesia, you may feel drowsy, weak, or nauseated for a short time after your procedure. Be sure to tell your nurse if you have any burning sensation in the perineum where the seeds were inserted, sweating, or other unusual symptoms.

Will I be in pain as a result of my radiation seeding treatment?

Most of the time you will not have severe pain. However, you might be uncomfortable. You may be given sleeping pills or other medication to relax you. If you feel you need pain medicine, be sure to let the radiation oncologist or urologist know. You may have a catheter in your bladder for a short time after the procedure, but you will probably be able to urinate the next day without a problem.

How long after the radiation seeding treatment will I be able to go back to work and my normal activities?

Usually you can go back to work and to your normal activities, such as exercising or walking, within a few days. Doctors advise that you not resume sexual activities for about four to six weeks.

Will I be impotent after radiation seeding treatments?

You may have some erection problems immediately following your treatment, but a large percentage of men who have had this treatment report that they are still able to have erections, although they may not be as firm as they were before treatment.

chapter 11

What Happens If I Choose Watchful Waiting?

> The idea of watchful waiting or careful observation as a treatment option may be frightening to you if you view all cancers as aggressive and fast growing. However, it is a known fact that the great majority of men with prostate cancer die *with* it rather than *from* it. The fact that the incidence of prostate cancer increases with age and that nearly all men over age 80 have signs of prostate cancer at autopsy gives a powerful argument for choosing this option if you are over 70 or if your cancer is a low-grade, well-differentiated, unaggressive, slow-growing one.

For some men, choosing the option of keeping the cancer under observation is a real choice. This does not mean that you can go home and forget about having to return for follow-up exams and repeated PSA tests. A number of factors—your general health, your family history, your age, the type of cancer, and your own mental attitude—must be taken into consideration.

When is watchful waiting a treatment option?

Watchful waiting (also referred to as deferred therapy, careful observation, and active surveillance) depends upon your age, your general health, the size of your cancer, and the type of cancer. It is important that you understand exactly what you are dealing with when you make the decision to wait and watch. Many studies show that some men with prostate cancer are not affected by it. However, there is a risk involved. If you make this choice based on the wrong assumptions and do not keep a close watch, it is likely that you may have to deal with an advanced case of prostate cancer if you live long enough.

What kind of risk am I taking by choosing watchful waiting?

Very little if you continue to be carefully monitored, you are assured that you have a low PSA, and your cancer is a low-grade, well-differentiated, unaggressive one. If this is the case, there is an 85 percent chance that you will **not** die from it within the next 10 years. After 10 years, the risk becomes higher.

Who might consider the watchful waiting route?

- Men with low-grade (T1a) and well-differentiated cancers.
- Men with low PSA levels.
- Men who are in their seventies or eighties with a limited long-term life expectancy.
- Men in their sixties and seventies who have other life-threatening health problems.

Who should not consider watchful waiting?

Younger men, ages 50 to 60, who have no life-threatening illness and expect to live a long time should consider having treatment for their prostate cancers. Moderately differentiated or undifferentiated cancers are usually biologically more aggressive, and treatment for men with those kinds of cancers is usually indicated.

QUESTIONS TO ASK ABOUT WATCHFUL WAITING

- **Is watchful waiting a possible option for me?**
- **Would you categorize my cancer as low grade and well differentiated? As slow growing and nonaggressive?**

"That last part of the physical exam, the digital, never was my favorite," says 59-year-old Cecil M. "Just the same, I'd never given it a second thought until the doctor called and told me I might have a problem." Thinking back on it, Cecil says he might have been naive, because he had been having some problems with urination but had chalked it up to age. "My problem was that I was told that I could watch and wait—and it just isn't my style. The doctor said I should come in every three months to have my PSA checked—and just not to worry about it meantime. My PSA right now is 3.5, up from 3 six months ago. I'm leaving on a one-month business trip out of the country, and I keep worrying that something might happen while I'm away. "

One doctor's comment on this was: Tell him to stop worrying and take his trip. One month won't make a difference. He can have the PSA done again when he comes back and see if it's elevated further. There's time to make a decision then.

- At what point will you suggest I have treatment?
- How will you monitor me if I choose watchful waiting?
- How often will you repeat the PSA?
- At what point do you consider the PSA sufficiently elevated to warrant treatment?
- Will my options at that point be different from what they are right now?

What are the results of studies that choose watchful waiting rather than treatment?

One randomized study of 95 men comparing radical prostatectomy in Stages I and II cancers did not show a significant difference in survival after 4 to 9 years. Another study of 828 men with clinically localized cancers had no treatment but were followed and given hormone therapy at the time when it appeared that the cancer had progressed. This study showed that the men with Grade 1 or 2 tumors had a survival rate of 87 percent after 12 years and that their expected survival was the same as that for other men of similar ages in the general population. However, there has been no large study that has compared watchful waiting with radical prostatectomy or radiation treatment. There is one study underway (PIVOT) that is comparing radical prostatectomy and watchful waiting, but it will be many years before the results are known (see Chapter 14).

How will the doctor monitor me if I choose to wait and watch?

You should probably see your doctor every four to six months. The doctor will check your PSA, do a digital exam, do a urinalysis to check for blood, and review your physical symptoms with you. Some men sometimes ask to have the PSA taken every month. This really is not necessary and can be counterproductive and disturbing, because the PSA can fluctuate from test to test. In addition, you will not need to repeat your ultrasound, bone scan, or biopsy unless there is a change. The PSA and digital exam should be adequate to monitor your condition. Usually, if the cancer is progressing, there will be an increase in the PSA over time. If this occurs, most doctors prefer to check the PSA two or three times over three or four months to be sure that the elevation in the PSA is more than just a normal fluctuation or a lab error. If the PSA continues to increase over time and there is a change in the digital exam, with the nodule becoming more pronounced or harder, then it may be necessary to decide on one of the forms of treatment. If the PSA remains stable, your doctor will probably suggest that you can lengthen the time between checkups.

At what point would treatment be considered?

There is no way, with present techniques, of knowing for sure what is the appropriate time to begin treatment just as there is no way of knowing for sure that the cancer is remaining confined to the prostate gland. Significant changes in the PSA and the digital exam may require a treatment review. Some studies show that if you live 10 years or more after diagnosis of cancer and you have not had any treatment, your odds of dying from prostate cancer may begin to increase.

Is it possible that my primary doctor will suggest watchful waiting and my urologist will recommend immediate treatment?

Conflicting advice from two physicians is not unusual. If this happens, it probably would be wise for you to get another opinion from another urologist who has no connection with the other physicians. Try to seek out someone who regularly deals with a large number of prostate cancer cases.

chapter 12

What Happens If I Have Cryosurgery?

Archeologists know that the use of ice as anesthesia for surgery was first described in about 3500 B.C. The cancer freezing concept has been studied since the 1850s. Surgeons have been using cryosurgery to treat skin cancers for years. But for harder-to-reach organs such as the prostate, freezing was a problem because it was not possible to see exactly how much tissue was being destroyed. When cryosurgery was first used in 1966, it was found that the inability to control the freezing caused damage to the urethra and often led to urinary problems because pieces of dead prostate tissue would slough off and plug up the urinary tract.

In the late 1980s, ultrasound imaging techniques provided new and easier ways to image anatomical structures inside the body. These imaging techniques allowed surgeons to reconsider the use of cryosurgery as a means of destroying cancerous tissue in the prostate. The development of new thin, easily positioned cryoprobes and a urethral warming device, which protects the urethra

(continued)

while the prostate gland is being frozen, has significantly reduced the complications originally reported in cryosurgery.

This treatment is controversial because it has not been evaluated over a sufficient period of time or been proven against radical prostatectomy and radiation therapy. Some physicians have been slow to endorse prostate cryosurgery because they feel there is a conflict of interest since the cryosurgical equipment is primarily available only through manufacturers with financial ties to some of the physicians using the equipment. The testing of prostate cryosurgery is underway in clinical studies, and many men are considering cryosurgery as another alternative in dealing with prostate cancer.

A number of men have chosen cryosurgery after considering other possible alternatives. Because of the relative simplicity of the treatment and the reduced costs and side effects, this treatment could become a preferred treatment for prostate cancer. However, at this time, the treatment has not be used long enough to determine how effective it is over the long term.

Long-term problems that can be expected after cryosurgery in a group of 100 men who had the procedure include:

Impotence	70–80
Incontinence	10
Incontinence with prior radiation	50
Blocked urethra	5–20

What is cryosurgery?

Cryosurgery, also sometimes referred to as cryotherapy or cryoablation, is the use of extreme cold to destroy cancer cells. Liquid nitrogen is circulated through cryoprobes, which are placed in contact with the tumor.

Who are the best candidates for cryosurgery?

Cryosurgery is being used to treat men with early-stage cancer that is confined to the prostate gland and the surrounding area, particularly when standard treatments such as surgery and radiation are unsuccessful or cannot be used. Clinical trials are being conducted with several groups of men:

- Men with Stage II prostate cancer who prefer not to have a radical prostatectomy or radiation therapy or who have risk factors that make other treatments not feasible for them.
- Men diagnosed with Stage III prostate cancer.

Can cryosurgery be used if I had radiation or radiation seeding and have a recurrence?

Cryosurgery is sometimes used to prevent progression of cancer in men who have had previous treatment with radiation.

Are there cases where cryosurgery should not be used?

Cryosurgery is not considered an effective treatment for prostate cancer that has spread to the lymph nodes or to distant parts of the body.

Who performs cryosurgery?

Because cryosurgery is a newer treatment for prostate cancer, the treatment is available in selected hospitals across the country. You will find a list of hospitals who have doctors who do cryosurgery in Chapter 16, Where to Get Help.

How is cryosurgery performed?

The liquid nitrogen or carbon dioxide is placed in a hollow metal probe that freezes and destroys unwanted or diseased tissue, which is then absorbed by the body over time. Probes are positioned directly into the prostate through the area between the anus and the base of scrotum.

Does cryosurgery involve surgery?

The surgery involves a small incision for insertion of the cryo-probe through the skin in the perineum. However, the treatment is considered a surgical procedure and takes two to three hours

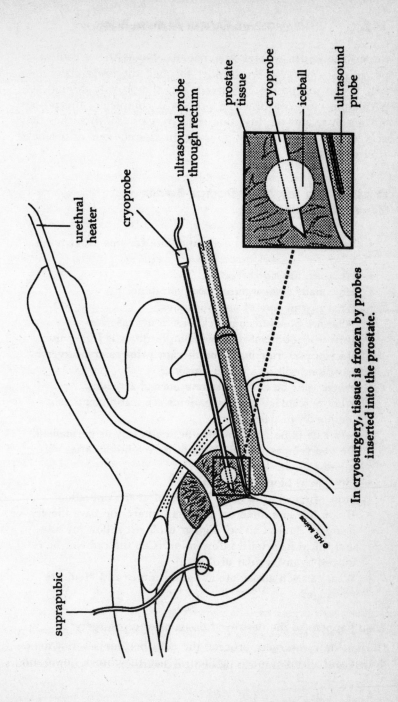

urethral heater

cryoprobe

ultrasound probe through rectum

suprapubic

prostate tissue

cryoprobe

iceball

ultrasound probe

In cryosurgery, tissue is frozen by probes inserted into the prostate.

© H.R. Malinac

to perform under general or spinal anesthesia. After a catheter is put in place to drain the bladder through the lower abdominal wall, probes are positioned directly into the prostate through the perineum. Once the freezing process is completed, the probes are removed and the insertion sites are closed with stiches that dissolve. Most men are able to leave the hospital one or two days after surgery.

QUESTIONS TO ASK YOUR DOCTOR BEFORE HAVING CRYOSURGERY

- Do you think I am a good candidate for this procedure? Why?
- What are the side effects?
- How many cryosurgeries have you done?
- What is your rate of complications?
- What are possible complications in my case?
- How will you manage these complications if I have them?
- Do you prescribe hormone therapy prior to cryosurgery?
- How long will I be in the hospital?
- When will I be able to resume normal activities?
- What percentage of your patients are incontinent? Is it temporary or permanent?
- Will I be impotent? Will this be temporary or permanent?
- Do you require your patients to have a biopsy after six months to check results? Why?
- How many biopsies do you do?
- How often will I need to see you after the operation?
- If you live in a different city than where you have the cryosurgery done: Can my regular urologist follow my case and will you forward information? Can the catheter be removed by my regular urologist?
- What can you advise me about insurance and Medicare coverage?

What happens to the destroyed tissue after cryosurgery?

During the cryosurgery process, the cells become severely dehydrated and shrink. Once engulfed by ice, they break down and are destroyed and frozen intracellularly. As melting occurs, the destruction continues and the capillaries supplying oxygen and other nutrients to the tumor are damaged beyond repair. Clotting and local tissue swelling and the invasion of the immune system's scavenger cells cause the destroyed tissue to be absorbed by the body. During the next weeks, the body's white blood cells engulf the dead cellular material, leaving behind normal, fibrous tissue. When examined on follow-up, what remains will be a shrunken, prostatic capsule, relatively free of glandular tissue.

How do I prepare for cryosurgery?

Before cryosurgery, you will be given specific instructions regarding diet and enemas. The enema will help clear your bowels so that the ultrasound will be clear.

What are the risks and side effects of cryosurgery?

The risks associated with cryosurgery are the same as those for any surgical procedure. There are side effects, although they may be less severe than those associated with surgery or radiation therapy. The urinary system may be affected. Incontinence and impotence can result from cryosurgery, although these side effects may be temporary. Present data show that 70 to 80 percent of men are impotent after cryosurgery.

What are the advantages of cryosurgery?

The advantages include a decrease in the incidence of serious complications, a short hospital stay, and the ability to repeat the procedure if needed. There is no abdominal incision, and bleeding complications are minimal. Cryosurgery is usually less expensive than other treatments and requires a shorter recovery time and a shorter hospital stay.

What are the disadvantages of cryosurgery?

The major disadvantage is the uncertainty regarding the long-term effectiveness of the treatment. If freezing is not carefully controlled, tissue near the rectal wall may be damaged, causing a fistula to develop between the rectum and urethra. Men who have undergone radiation therapy for prostate cancer are at greatest risk for this complication. In addition, because the effectiveness of the technique is still being assessed, insurance coverage problems may arise.

"I was not about to give up my sex life," says Jim, an early retiree who spends his time sketching and helping at the local art center. "So, when I found out that my Gleason score of 5 wasn't good news, I told the doctor that I would not consider surgery. I have two good friends who went that route and have lived to regret it. He was upset with me but made arrangements for me to see a radiation oncologist. I went through my six weeks of radiation without too many problems except some diarrhea. Two years later on my 63rd birthday, my doctor told me my PSA was up again.

"During the last couple of years I've done a lot of thinking and a lot of talking with other men who've had the same problem. I decided to go for a consultation at a clinic where they are conducting clinical trials on cryosurgery. They told me that even though I'd already had radiation, I was a perfect candidate for cryosurgery. I've just had it done, and I was surprised at how I sailed through the treatment. Except for the fact that when I got home I had a catheter in my abdomen, I was able to be up and around. Recovery took a little longer than was advertised, but after about six weeks I'm back to normal, although I still have urgency problems with urination but no dribbling."

Will I still be able to have erections after cryosurgery?

Because the experience with cryosurgery is still limited, the results are not fully known. Some men report that they are able to continue to have erections. About 20 to 30 percent of men who had erections prior to cryosurgery have regained this ability within six months to a year after treatment. It is possible that this rate may increase over time, because nerves can regenerate following freezing.

Will I be incontinent after cryosurgery?

Incontinence has been reported in 1.5 percent of men who had cryosurgery and had not had prior radiation. Those who had prior radiation had about a 50 percent chance of having some degree of incontinence following the procedure. Urinary control may improve over time for most of these men but may not return completely.

What other problems can occur following cryosurgery?

Tissue sloughing may occur when pieces of prostate tissue break off and fall into the bladder or urethra, blocking the flow of urine. This has been minimized by the warming of the urethra. Tissue sloughing usually corrects itself without the need for further treatment. Fistulas, or holes, can develop between the urinary and gastrointestinal tract, which may later require a surgical operation to repair. Irritation to the bladder or urethra is another common side effect that causes problems with urination, such as the need to urinate with little warning, pain with urination, and a burning sensation.

Should men with large prostates consider cryosurgery?

Cryosurgery works best when the prostate gland is about 40 grams or less in size. At some centers, physicians prescribe three to four months of total hormone blockage using both monthly shots of luteinizing hormone-releasing hormone and flutamide to shrink the gland before doing the cryosurgery.

How long will I be in the hospital?

Usually one or two days. Most men are able to get up and move about the afternoon after cryosurgery, eat their evening meal, and leave the next day. A small tube just below the navel will be in place and will be left in place for about 10 to 14 days. (You may find sweatpants are more comfortable than regular trousers while the tube is in place.) This suprapubic tube is placed in the bladder as a safety release valve for when you try to urinate through the penis for the first time. Antibiotics are usually prescribed.

When can I go back to doing my regular activities?

You can usually go back to work or resume your regular activities within a week or two.

Is there pain involved with the procedure?

There is tenderness in the area between the anus and the testicles at the point where the cryoprobes are inserted. There usually is some swelling of the testicles. As with all such treatments, there is some discomfort, but most men do not require pain medication. Healing is usually complete within three months.

Does it hurt to have the suprapubic catheter removed?

Usually there is no pain involved when the catheter is removed.

Can the cryosurgery procedure be repeated if I have a recurrence?

One of the benefits of cryosurgery is that it can be repeated if the first procedure does not eliminate the cancer. The physician may selectively freeze areas where recurrence occurs.

What is the cost of the procedure and does insurance or Medicare cover costs?

The cost of cryosurgery, hospitalization, and the physician's fee can range from $12,000 to $15,000. Not every insurance company covers cryosurgery, and it appears that reimbursement is presently being made on a case-by-case basis. Insurers who pay for the procedure have cited the facts of shortened length of hospitalization and lower costs as reasons for coverage. Insurers who have not paid cite the need for more published data. Medicare doesn't usually reimburse the costs. However, as more and more men are having cryosurgery and as more surgeons and hospitals are providing this treatment, it is expected that modifications will be made.

Where is cryosurgery being performed?

Over 100 hospitals in the United States are performing cryosurgery. Some are conducting clinical trials on the procedure, while others are doing the procedure without being involved in clinical trials. A listing of centers where cryosurgery is being performed can be found in Chapter 16. If you are interested in enrolling in cryosurgery clinical trials, see Chapter 14.

What is available to me if I need additional treatment after my cryosurgery?

Besides being able to have cryosurgery again, you also can be treated with hormones, surgery, radiation, or watchful waiting.

chapter 13

What Happens If I Have Hormone Treatment?

> For years, scientists have known that prostate cancer cells depend on male sex hormones for their growth. Like breast cancer, prostate cancer is sensitive to hormones. These hormones stimulate the growth of prostate cancer cells. When certain hormones are eliminated from the body, the cancer may stop growing and become inactive for a period of time—from 1 to 10 years. The purpose of hormone therapy is to lower levels of testosterone. Although it is not a curative treatment, hormone therapy is often used to treat prostate cancer. The treatment may be given before or after prostatectomy or radiation therapy and sometimes before radiation seeding or cryosurgery.

How does hormone treatment work?

You may hear several different terms used to describe hormone treatment—combination hormone therapy, androgens, complete hormone blockage, complete adrogen blockage, and ablation. Because prostate cancer is sensitive to hormones, it has been found that eliminating testosterone from the body deprives the cancer of this hormone and usually prevents it from growing. Testosterone is controlled by a pituitary hormone called luteinizing hormone. Two drugs, goserelin acetate and leuprolide acetate, affect the pituitary gland's response to the chemical signal to make testosterone and lower the testosterone to the same low levels as if your testicles had been removed. However, some testosterone may be produced by your adrenal glands. Flutamide has been found to block the effects of the remaining hormone.

How is hormone treatment used in treating prostate cancer?

Hormonal manipulation—either with hormone drugs or with the surgical removal of the testicles—is being used in a number of different ways in treating prostate cancer.

- It may be used when the cancer is localized but is in an advanced stage.
- It may be the primary treatment in older men when it is felt that radiation or surgery is too risky or inappropriate.
- It is sometimes used before cryosurgery or radiation seeding or before or after surgery or radiation to reduce the prostate size or to keep the tumor from growing.
- It may be the treatment of choice if the cancer has spread or returned after previous treatment.

What are the different types of hormone treatments used for prostate cancer?

A number of different therapies are available. These include:

- Luteinizing hormone-releasing hormone agonist (LHRH).
- Antiandrogen.
- Orchiectomy (removal of testicles).
- Estrogen (diethylstilbestrol, DES).

QUESTIONS TO ASK YOUR DOCTOR ABOUT HORMONE TREATMENT

- What kind of hormone treatment do you suggest for me?
- Why are you suggesting this type of hormone treatment?
- How long will it be before we know whether this treatment works for me?
- How often will you check my PSA level to see how well the hormone treatment is working?
- What are the possible side effects?
- Will I get hot flashes?
- What is the cost of the treatment?
- Do you ever advise your patients to have an orchiectomy? Do you do the surgery? What are the risks? What are the advantages and disadvantages?
- Do you advise having hormone therapy before or after surgery or radiation? Before radiation seeding or cryosurgery?
- How do you usually treat bone metastases?
- How much does it cost? Is it covered by insurance or Medicare?

What are luteinizing hormone-releasing hormone agonists, often referred to as LHRHs (Lupron, Depo Lupron, and Zoladex)?

LHRH suppresses testicular androgen and is the normal brain hormone that controls the secretion of luteinizing hormone from the pituitary gland, responsible for stimulating the secretion of male hormones by the testes. The natural hormone LHRH is secreted by the brain in minute amounts and successive pulses of the hormone are released approximately once every 90 minutes. When LHRH was first discovered, it was hoped that it would be useful for increasing fertility and gonadal functions. Unexpectedly, when it was copied in the laboratory and made 100 to 300 times more potent than the natural hormone, it was found that it had the opposite effect, blocking the effects of the natural hormones. Therefore, LHRH is now being used to inhibit testicular functions. Several forms being made in the laboratory are being used, including the leuprolides (Lupron and Depo Lupron) and goserelin (Zoladex).

"My son is a doctor, so when I found out my PSA was in the questionable range I called him, thinking I'd let him guide me in making a decision about what to do. Much to my surprise there were so many options and so much controversy about the various treatments that I set out on my own discovery adventure, and I've turned up some pretty interesting stuff—from cryosurgery to hyperthermia. I'm now on a six-month hormonal regimen to shrink the cancer and I still haven't made a firm decision about what to do next."

How is the LHRH treatment given?

Lupron is usually given as a monthly injection in the muscle of the buttock. **Zoladex** is a pellet that is injected under the surface of the skin somewhere on the abdominal wall. (Longer-acting versions of these medications are being developed, which will allow injections that will last several months.) The shot stimulates a short burst of testosterone, which your body interprets as having too much testosterone, causing the body to shut down the hormone production. In some cases, during the period of increased testosterone levels, there can be problems, such as increased bone pain (flare). The addition of antiandrogen helps block tumor flare in the first few weeks or months of treatment, after which the antiandrogen is often discontinued. This treatment is expensive and causes loss of sexual desire and potency. It costs about $400 to $500 per month for life.

How are antiandrogens used?

Androgens are hormones secreted by the testes and adrenal glands, which are necessary for the development of male sexual characteristics and function. Antiandrogens reduce or eliminate the activity of these androgens. There is some evidence that this male hormone also plays a role in stimulating prostate cancer. **Flutamide**, which is sold under the brand name **Eulexin**, is a synthetic nonsteroidal antiandrogen that blocks the cells' ability to absorb any hormone, producing what is called total androgen blockage, and thus blocks any androgens produced by the adrenal glands not suppressed by LHRH treatment. Tablets are usually taken three times a day and the cost is $250 to $300 per month for life. A newer nonsteroidal antiandrogen is **bicalutamide**, sold under the brand name **Casodex**. Because antiandrogens can stimulate breast growth, a small amount of radiation is usually given to the breasts before treatment begins to help keep breasts from enlarging.

How is flutamide used in prostate cancer?

This drug has been used alone as well as in combination with LHRH or immunotherapy in an attempt to suppress tumor growth in prostate cancer. In many cases, when used alone, sexual potency can be preserved. It is effective but less so than LHRH. Flutamide and nilutamide are sometimes used together or in combination with orchiectomy in Stage IV cancers to produce bone pain relief and slow the progression of the cancer.

What are the side effects of flutamide?

Side effects are generally limited to mild diarrhea and breast enlargement, but liver poisoning can sometimes occur. The liver usually recovers when the drug is stopped. Occasionally when flutamide is stopped after you have been taking it for a long period there may be a drop in your PSA levels.

What is Casodex (bicalutamide)?

Casodex is a new drug, recently approved by the Food and Drug Administration, which is similar to flutamide but has the advantage of requiring only a single daily dose. It is a nonsteroidal antiandrogen often used with LHRH. When given with LHRH, it achieves maximal androgen blockade by preventing any remaining testosterone from binding to receptor sites in prostate cancer cells.

What are the side effects of Casodex?

Hot flashes are experienced by about half of those taking the pill. Constipation, back pain, lack of strength, pelvic pain, nausea, and diarrhea have also been reported.

How does estrogen therapy (DES) work?

Estrogen is a synthetic female hormone that reduces or eliminates the body's production of testosterone. DES, in the form of a daily

pill, is sometimes prescribed, although this treatment is used less
often now that alternative treatments are available. There are side
effects to this treatment, such as breast enlargement or tenderness, nausea, vomiting, loss of libido, impotence, and blood clots.
This form of treatment is not appropriate for men who have a
history of heart disease or embolism.

What is intermittent therapy?

Hormone therapy is sometimes used on an intermittent basis. It
is first used until your PSA drops down to its lowest level and
stabilizes. Then it is withdrawn. When the PSA level starts to climb
again, the hormone therapy is started again. Therapy is then continued until the PSA drops down again. This treatment is being
studied in clinical trials.

When is an orchiectomy used for prostate cancer?

Most men are appalled at the thought of an operation on their
testicles. The idea of being castrated is emotionally a difficult issue. Yet orchiectomy, the removal of the testicles, has been used
for many years to control prostate cancers. The spread of prostate
cancer can often be controlled by removing the testicles—the natural source of the male sex hormone. Removal of both testicles
is technically called a bilateral orchiectomy. This procedure,
which is considered a low-risk operation, eliminates the major
source of testosterone. Without this hormone, the growth of prostate cancer cells slows down. Men who have had the operation
report that there is little or no pain except for some possible
swelling, bruising, or soreness immediately after the procedure
that lasts a few days.

How is the orchiectomy operation done?

The operation consists of the removal of both testicles through a
small incision, leaving the scrotum intact. It is usually performed
as an outpatient procedure, done under anesthesia with absorb-
able stitches.

Is an orchiectomy the same as castration?

Orchiectomy and castration both mean that the testicles are removed.

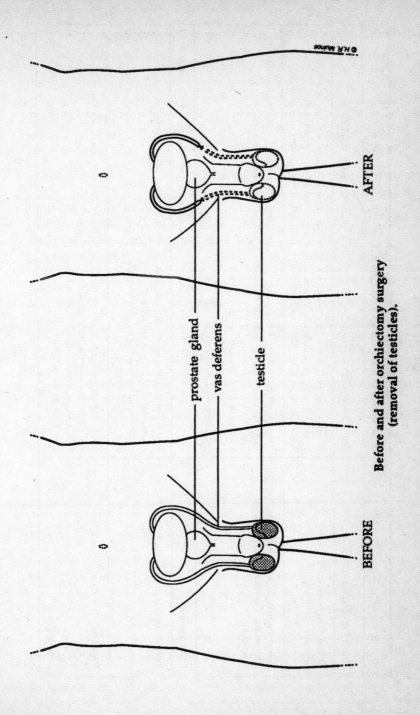

prostate gland

vas deferens

testicle

BEFORE

AFTER

Before and after orchiectomy surgery (removal of testicles).

© H.R. Muñoz

HORMONE TREATMENTS

TYPE OF TREATMENT	PROS AND CONS	POSSIBLE SIDE EFFECTS
LHRH (Lupron/Depo Lupron/Zoladex)	Monthly injection. Achieves same effect as orchiectomy surgery. Sometimes used with flutamide. Cost: $400–$500/month for life.	May cause hot flashes, breast tenderness, reduced sex drive, possible flare-up immediately after start of treatment.
Antiandrogens, flutamide (Eulexin), **nilutamide, Casodex, total androgen blockage**	Given in pill form three times a day. Radiation usually given to breasts. Can be added to other treatment if PSA levels rise. Cost: $250–$300/month for life. (Casodex is given in pill form once a day. Cost: about $270–$500/month for life.)	Diarrhea, hot flashes, reduced sex drive. Occasional liver problems.
Ketoconazole		Impotence, nail changes, liver problems.
Orchiectomy (removal of testicles)	Simple outpatient surgery, immediate drop in testosterone levels. Is considered emasculating by many men. Not reversible. Cost: $2,000–3,000	Hot flashes, breast tenderness, impotence.
Estrogen (DES)	Given daily in pill form. Low cost but high risk. There are other safer alternatives. Testosterone levels drop in 30–60 days. Cost: $10–30/month for life.	Higher doses can cause strokes or blood clots.

How effective is an orchiectomy?

As a treatment for dropping the testosterone level, an orchiectomy achieves the desired goal quickly and efficiently. The testosterone level drops to zero within the first 12 hours after the operation. If there is bone pain caused by cancer, it usually also disappears. The one-time cost of the operation makes it much less expensive than the cost of the other alternatives, and it is usually covered by insurance.

TREATING BONE METASTASES

How are bone metastases caused by prostate cancer treated?

Eighty to 85 percent of prostate cancer metastases are found in the bone. The other 10 to 15 percent are in soft tissue including lymph nodes, liver, and lung. For those with bone metastases, the treatment recommended is usually orchiectomy with or without antiandrogens or LHRH with or without flutamide or estrogens. There are clinical trials underway for neutron/photon radiation, chemotherapy, and other hormone treatments.

What other kinds of treatment are available for bone metastases?

If the metastatic cancer is confined to one area, external-beam radiation may be used. Where there are more widespread problems, investigation is underway with bone-seeking radioisotopes and radioactive monoclonal antibodies. Strontium-89, sometimes referred to as Metastron, is an injectable form of radioactive isotope that is sometimes used for treatment of painful multiple bone metastases. Another radioisotope, tin-117 DPTA, is being tested to treat bone pain.

How does strontium-89 work?

Strontium-89 is injected and goes directly to the sites of metastatic bone disease, where, like calcium, it is absorbed into the bones. The injection contains small amounts of a specially selected form of radioactive strontium, chosen because almost all of its radioactivity is absorbed, allowing it to deliver therapy precisely where it is needed. A single injection generally provides pain relief for an average of six months and has minimal effect on normal bone and surrounding tissues. The effects of strontium-89 are confined within your body. Other people cannot receive the effects of radiation through bodily contact with you. However, for the first week after injection, strontium-89 will be present in your blood and urine, and your doctor will discuss simple precautions that should be taken. Stronium-89 is not recommended for patients with cancer that does not involve bone.

What are the side effects of strontium-89 (Metastron)?

Some people experience a mild facial flushing immediately after injection. This may happen when the medication is administered too quickly (in 30 seconds rather than in one or two minutes). Some people have a mild but temporary increase in pain several days after the injection that may last for two or three days. Doctors usually prescribe an increase in painkillers until the pain is under control. After approximately one or two weeks, the pain begins to diminish, and relief continues for up to six months. You may be advised to reduce the dose of pain medications gradually. Eventually, you may not need painkillers at all. You can eat and drink normally. There may be a slight fall in your blood cell count. Your doctor will probably ask you to have routine periodic blood tests. Repeated dosages can be given if the doctor feels this is the most appropriate treatment.

chapter 14

What about Other Treatments?

> In the course of researching this book, we came across a variety of treatments for prostate cancer that you may have heard or read about. Some of these treatments have a sound scientific basis and are presently being tested in clinical trials on men with recurrent and metastatic prostate cancer. Some are being promoted by health food stores and by people involved in alternative medicine. Some are totally unproven, perhaps even absurd. We have separated those that are undergoing clinical trials from those that fall into the unproven area to give you a way of understanding the difference so that you can make your own decisions on how you want to proceed.

CLINICAL TRIALS

Some specific clinical trials testing different treatments have been discussed in Chapters 8 through 13. Many different kinds of trials are being conducted by doctors across the United States. This chapter deals with clinical trials that have not been covered in previous chapters.

WHAT YOU NEED TO KNOW ABOUT CLINICAL TRIALS

- Clinical trials (also called investigational or experimental treatment) remain the critical link between researchers with microscopes and test tubes and the transfer of new techniques to patients.
- Each clinical trial is designed to answer a set of research questions. You need to fit into the guidelines for a trial—usually a certain type and stage of cancer and certain health status—to be eligible to take part.
- The new treatment is often based on a standard treatment, that is, the state-of-the-art treatment now being used.
- There are safeguards built into the trial to protect you. For example, a special review board looks at the study to see that it is well designed and that potential risks to patients are reasonable in relation to the potential benefits. You usually have more tests and will be monitored more frequently than a regular patient.

QUESTIONS TO ASK BEFORE PARTICIPATING IN A CLINICAL TRIAL FOR TREATMENT

- What is the purpose of the clinical trial?
- What are the possible benefits?
- Who is sponsoring it? (NCI? A major cancer center? A pharmaceutical firm?)
- Why do the doctors who designed the study believe that the treatment being studied may be better than the one now being used?
- Who will be giving the treatment?
- How long will I be in the study?
- What kinds of tests are involved? Are they in addition to the tests that would normally be done? Will I have to pay for them?

- What will the treatment consist of? How does it differ from the standard treatment?
- Will I be hospitalized?
- What are the possible side effects or risks of the new treatment? How do they compare with the standard treatment?
- How does the treatment I would receive in this study compare with the other choices in terms of possible outcomes, side effects, time involved, cost to me, and quality of life?
- How could the study affect my daily life?
- Can I stop my participation at any time? What happens if I do?
- Will I have to pay for the treatment? Does the study provide any of it free of charge? Will insurance routinely pay for treatment?
- Does the study include long-term follow-up care? How often will that be and what will it consist of?

CHEMOTHERAPY AND BIOLOGICALS

Is chemotherapy used to treat prostate cancer?

There are many clinical trials being conducted with chemotherapy drugs, usually in combination. Most of them have not worked well when used as the main treatment. However, many times they are used as a secondary treatment to slow the growth of the tumor, especially in Stage IV or recurrent prostate cancer or as an approach to control pain. In addition, some new drugs are showing promise and are presently in clinical trials.

Are biologicals being used to treat prostate cancer?

There are some biologicals being tested. Biologicals are one of the newest developments in cancer treatment—using substances to trigger the body's own defenses against cancer. These substances boost, direct, or restore many of the normal defenses of the body. Many of them occur naturally in the body, whereas others are made in the laboratory. Doctors are just beginning to experiment with ways of combining various biologicals with each other and with standard treatments for more effective use.

What substances are used in the biological area for prostate cancer?

The substances in clinical trials for prostate cancer include monoclonal antibodies, interferons, tumor growth factors, and gene therapy.

What are monoclonal antibodies?

A *monoclonal antibody* is a substance that can find and attach to a specific protein on cancer cells. Monoclonal antibodies are produced in the body in small quantities. However, they can be produced in a laboratory in large quantities and introduced into the body to hone in on target cancer cells. They have potential in the prevention, detection, and treatment of cancer.

Are monoclonal antibodies being used in treating prostate cancer?

There are some clinical trials using monoclonal antibodies to deliver anticancer drugs directly to the cancer cells, thereby increasing the attack on those cells while causing less damage to normal healthy cells.

What are some of the agents linked to the monoclonal antibodies?

The agents linked to the antibodies include radioisotopes, chemotherapy drugs, biological agents, tumor growth factors, and interferon.

What are tumor growth factors?

Tumor growth factors, which are also called cytokines, colony-stimulating factors, or hematopoietic growth factors, are naturally occurring substances that stimulate the bone marrow to produce white and red blood cells and platelets. Growth factors can enable patients to tolerate larger doses of chemotherapy.

How are growth factors given?

Growth factors are usually given either intravenously or subcutaneously (under the skin). Sometimes patients are able to give them to themselves after instruction by a nurse.

What is interferon?

Interferon, discovered in 1975, is a cytokine, a protein that helps to regulate the immune system. Interferons used in cancer treat-

SELECTED CHEMOTHERAPY DRUGS AND BIOLOGICALS BEING TESTED FOR ADVANCED PROSTATE CANCER

Name	Possible Side Effects
CPT-11 (Irinotecan, camptothecin-11)	Low blood counts, anemia, diarrhea, nausea and vomiting, mouth sores, constipation, flushing, cramping, loss of hair, skin rash, fever, shortness of breath, tearing.
Cyclophosphamide (Cytoxan, Neosar, Endoxan)	Nausea, vomiting, loss of appetite, hair loss. Blood in urine, pain when urinating, black tarry stools, fever, chills, nasal stuffiness and sore throat, cough and shortness of breath, dizziness, confusion, fast heartbeat, sterility (may be temporary), skin darkening, metallic taste during injection, blurred vision, cataract, second cancers (leukemia, bladder).
Doxorubicin (Adriamycin, Rubex, Adriamycin RDF, PFS, or MDV)	Nausea and vomiting, red urine (usually lasts one or two days after each dose), hair loss, loss of appetite, heart problems. Mouth sores; darkening of soles, palms, or nails; fever; chills; sore throat; diarrhea; eye problems; fast or irregular heartbeat; shortness of breath; pain in joint, side, or stomach; burning pain at injection site. May reactivate skin reactions from past radiation.
Interferon alpha-n1 (Wellferon), Interferon alpha-n2A, 2B (Roferon, Intron A), Interferon alpha-2C (Berofor)	Fever, chills, and sweats (usually occur in 1–2 hours; last less than 18 hours), tiredness, lack of energy, loss of appetite, change in taste, muscle pain, headaches, sleeplessness, depression, visual disturbances, tremor, seizures, agitation, anxiety, dizziness, mild nausea and vomiting, diarrhea, gas, constipation, mild hair loss, skin rash and dryness, burning at injection site.

(continued)

SELECTED CHEMOTHERAPY DRUGS AND BIOLOGICALS BEING TESTED FOR ADVANCED PROSTATE CANCER *(cont.)*

NAME	POSSIBLE SIDE EFFECTS
Interferon gamma-1B (Actimmune)	Headache, fever, chills, diarrhea, nausea and vomiting, stomach pain, loss of appetite, dizziness, confusion, disorientation, hallucinations, seizures, tiredness, night sweats, shortness of breath, heart problems.
Mitomycin (Mutamycin, Mytomycin C)	Nausea and vomiting, loss of appetite, burning pain at injection site, fever, chills, and sore throat. Hair loss, fatigue and tiredness, diarrhea, mouth sores, blurred vision, blood in urine, numbness or tingling in fingers and toes, purple-colored bands on nails, skin rash, kidney or lung problems.
Mitoxantrone (Mitoxantrone hydrochloride, Novantrone, DHAD, DHAQ, NSC-301739).	Nausea and vomiting (usually can be prevented with antinausea medicine), mouth sores, hair loss (usually mild), blue-green urine (may last for 24 to 48 hours). Diarrhea, abdominal pain, skin rash, dry skin, chest pain, problems with breathing, headache, liver problems, blue streaking in and around vein.
Suramin (antrypol, Bayer 205, Germanin, Moranyl, Naganol, Fourneau 309, NSC-34936)	Nausea, vomiting, salty or metallic taste in mouth, anemia, constipation, skin rash, blood in urine, weakness in face muscles, eye problems (increased tears, blurred vision), fever, chills, and sore throat.

Drug	Side Effects
Tamoxifen (Nolvadex)	Nausea and vomiting, loss of appetite, hot flashes, bone and tumor pain, visual changes, skin rash and itchiness, dizziness, loss of hair, depression, light-headedness, confusion, fluid retention, headache, anemia, swelling of legs.
Taxol (Paclitaxel)	Anemia; hair loss (usually 14–21 days after treatment starts); heat flushes; shoulder, muscle, and joint pain; mouth sores (occur 3 to 7 days after first dose, get better 5 to 7 days later). Chest, stomach, or leg pain; fever; chills; sore throat; burning sensation in feet; loss of feeling in hands and feet; mild nausea and vomiting; diarrhea; fatigue; headache; alterations in taste; pain at injection site.
Topotecon (Hycamptamine, SNC-609699)	Headache, fatigue, weight loss, tiredness, low blood counts, anemia, nausea, vomiting, diarrhea, loss of weight, constipation, abdominal pain, hair loss, skin rash, acne, fever blisters, high blood pressure, rapid heartbeat, dizziness, light-headedness, numbness in fingers or toes, fever.
Vinblastine (Velban, Velsar, Alkaban AQ)	Decreased ability to make red and white blood cells and platelets. Nausea and vomiting; hair loss; mouth sores; loss of reflexes; fever; chills; sore throat; shortness of breath; burning pain, redness, or swelling at injection site; severe constipation; diarrhea; skin rash (sensitive to sun) and itching; mental depression; headache; pain in jaw, joints, bones, muscles, back, or limbs; pain in testicles; double vision; drooping eyelids.

ment are made naturally by the body when cells are stimulated by an agent, such as a virus, or produced synthetically in a laboratory by putting some interferons into bacteria and cultivating a large quantity of them.

Are there different kinds of interferons?

There are three groups of interferons: alpha, beta, and gamma. It appears that alpha and beta interferons are made by virtually all white blood cells. Gamma interferon is made only by T cells (a type of white blood cell processed in the thymus gland) and large granulocytes (a white blood cell made in the bone marrow). Gamma interferon is more powerful in its effect on the immune system than alpha or beta interferon.

Is interferon used alone in cancer treatment?

Interferon seems to be more effective when it is used with chemotherapy drugs or other biological agents.

Is anyone studying why prostate cancer seems to run in some families?

Men who have a close relative, such as a father or brother, with prostate cancer have a greater chance of developing prostate cancer themselves and of passing the genes for the disease on to their sons or grandsons. Several cancer centers are interviewing high-risk families, and collecting blood samples for analysis to determine the link of specific genes to prostate cancer. One new study—the Prostate Cancer Genetic Research Study (PROGRESS) is enrolling families with several men in them with prostate cancer. The men must be from the same side of the family but the relationship can be from either the mother's or father's side. They must be blood relatives.

How can I join the Prostate Cancer Genetic Research Study?

Your family may be eligible if you have three or more men who are related by blood who have been diagnosed with prostate cancer and at least two of these men are living. You will be asked to fill out a short questionnaire and have a blood sample taken. You will not need to have a physical exam or travel to be in the study. Family members, whether or not they have prostate cancer, including both men and women, will be asked to participate. You can get more information by calling 1-800-777-3035.

Are there any prostate prevention trials underway?
There are two:

1. The Prostrate Cancer Prevention Trial, to evaluate whether taking the drug Proscar (finasteride) for seven years will prevent prostate cancer from developing in men. This study is enrolling 18,000 men ages 55 and older, half of whom will receive finasteride each day for seven years and half of whom receive a placebo (an inactive pill that looks like finasteride).

2. The Prostate, Lung, Colorectal and Ovarian Cancer Screening Trial, to determine whether the widespread use of certain screening tests to detect these cancers will save lives. This test will study digital rectal exam and PSA (prostate), chest x-ray (lung), flexible sigmoidoscope (colorectum), and physical exam of the ovaries, CA-125, and transvaginal ultrasound (ovary). Doctors expect to enroll 148,000 men and women between the ages of 55 and 74 at 10 medical centers across the country.

What is the PIVOT clinical trial?

This randomized trial includes older men with early prostate cancer—that is, men whose cancer is only in the prostate. The men are being divided into two groups. One group is treated with a radical prostatectomy, and the other group is given watchful waiting—that is, no treatment but close and consistent follow-up. The PIVOT (Prostate Cancer Intervention Versus Observation Trial) study is designed to determine whether surgery is better than no surgery. Because this study will do long-term follow-up, it will be many years before the results are determined. This study is controversial, because it does not have a similar group that is being treated with radiation therapy.

CHEMOTHERAPY IMPLANTS

Are chemotherapy implants being tested?

An implant that releases 5-fluorouracil, a chemotherapy drug, is presently undergoing testing. The implant is injected directly into the prostate tumor, where it releases the drug for up to 48 hours and then self-destructs. Clinical trials are underway.

RADIATION

Is hormone blockage used in addition to radiation?

For men with Stage B2 and C prostate cancer, a trial is in progress to verify previous studies that used Zoladex plus flutamide for two months prior to radiation and with the continuation of androgen blockage during radiation. Original studies showed that this treatment gave superior local control (84 percent versus 71 percent).

What is high-LET radiation?

Neutron beams, heavy ions, and negative pi-mesons (pions) are known as high-LET (linear energy transfer) radiation. Facilities for high-LET radiation are limited at this time. Clinical trials have shown there are some advantages to this type of radiation, but the cost of the facilities and the sophistication of the personnel needed to carry it out presently restricts this treatment to selected referral centers for carefully selected patients.

Are there any new types of particle radiation being tested?

There are several new types that are being tested in clinical trials, including fast neutrons, deuterons, helium in beams, and negative pi-mesons. Most of these have limited application and are very costly. Their use is presently confined to a small number of cancer patients in clinical research studies.

Is heavy-ion treatment being conducted in the United States?

The heavy-ion accelerator at the Lawrence Berkeley Laboratory in Berkeley, California, that had treated some 400 patients since the 1970s was closed in 1993. It had been built mainly for high-energy physics. The first large accelerator in the world dedicated solely to cancer treatment, located outside of Tokyo, has been treating patients. There are plans to use a heavy-ion accelerator in Germany, and a cooperative European accelerator is also being built. In the United States, proton-beam treatment is being used instead of heavy ions.

Where is proton-beam radiation being done?

Two places in the United States have proton-beam accelerators for patient treatment: the Massachusetts General Hospital in Boston and Loma Linda University Medical Center in Los Angeles.

HYPERTHERMIA

What is hyperthermia?

Heat has been used in various ways for treating ailments since before the days of Hippocrates. Scientists think that exposing tissue to high temperatures may shrink tumors by damaging cells or depriving them of substances they need to live. Local (applying heat to a small area such as a tumor), regional (heating an organ or a limb), and whole-body hyperthermia are being studied.

How is the heating done?

External and internal heating devices can be used. For local hyperthermia, the area may be heated externally with high-frequency waves. Or it may be heated internally with a sterile probe, such as thin, heated wires or hollow tubes filled with warm water, implanted microwave antennae, radiofrequency electrodes, or laser implants that emit very high frequency sound waves. In regional hyperthermia, magnets and devices that produce high energy are placed over the region to be heated or the area is treated with perfusion—the patient's blood is removed, heated, and then pumped into the region that is to be heated internally. Whole-body heating uses warm-water blankets, hot wax, inductive coils (like those in electric blankets), or thermal chambers. There are clinical trials of this treatment method being conducted.

How can I find out about the specific clinical treatment trials being done for prostate cancer?

There are a number of ways you can proceed. First of all, explore the possibilities with your doctors. Get opinions from other cancer specialists. Go to or call a comprehensive cancer center if there is one in your area (see Chapter 16). Call the Cancer Information Service (1-800-4-CANCER) and ask the information specialists the questions you have about possible clinical treatment trials being offered for your stage of prostate cancer. You can also request that the Cancer Information Service do a PDQ search for clinical trials that pertain to your stage of prostate cancer.

Will my insurance company or health care plan pay for my treatment if I am on a clinical trial?

This is an important question you need to ask the doctor before you decide whether or not you are going to participate in a clinical trial. There are some agreements being signed between the health care payers and major institutions to allow cancer patients to be treated with these investigational, state-of-the-art treatments. The National Cancer Institute and the Department of Defense, for instance, have agreed to allow patients who use TRICARE/ CHAMPUS (the health program of the Department of Defense for members of the armed forces, their families, and others entitled to this health program) to participate in clinical treatment trials sponsored by the National Cancer Institute. The treatment can be given in the more than 2,000 medical centers around the country that conduct trials sponsored by the institute to test promising treatments for cancer (see Chapter 16).

What is PDQ?

PDQ is a data-based treatment information system supported by the National Cancer Institute. PDQ offers state-of-the-art treatment statements, compiled and updated monthly by panels of the country's leading cancer specialists, giving the range of effective treatment options that represent the best available therapy for a specific type or stage of cancer. PDQ also gives the latest information on clinical treatment trials being offered around the country for each type and stage of cancer. It is a ready reference, with over 1,000 active trials, that is updated monthly by review boards composed of cancer specialists.

What do I need to know in order to have a PDQ search of clinical trials for my kind of cancer?

If you call the Cancer Information Service and request a PDQ search, you will be asked a series of questions to determine the information needed to complete the search for you:

- Whether or not you are currently receiving treatment. (In some cases, if you are already being treated, you may not be eligible for clinical trials.)
- Whether you are interested in participating in a clinical trial.
- Whether you are able or willing to travel to a participating center and how far you are willing to travel for treatment.
- The primary site of your cancer, the stage, and if possible the cell type and grade.
- The site of metastases, if any.
- What previous treatments you have had, type of treatment, when and where, including the names of drugs previously received and when.
- Major medical conditions that might preclude participation.

Can I be treated at the Clinical Center at the National Institutes of Health?

The National Institutes of Health, the federal government's agency for medical research, has a medical research center and hospital—the Warren Grant Magnuson Clinical Center, located in Bethesda, Maryland, just outside of Washington, D.C. The hospital portion of the Clinical Center, with room for 540 patients, is especially designed for medical research. The number of beds available for a particular project and the length of the waiting list of qualified patients are important in determining whether and when you can be admitted. Research on a particular disease may allow only one or two patients to be studied at any given time.

How are patients selected for treatment at the Clinical Center?

You can be treated at the Clinical Center only if your case fits into a research project. Each project is designed to answer scientific questions and has specific medical eligibility requirements. For this reason you must be referred by your own doctor, who can supply the Clinical Center with the needed medical information, such as your diagnosis and details of your medical history. If your doctor feels that you might benefit by participating in a cancer research study at NIH, the doctor should call the National Cancer Institute's public inquiries office at 301-496-5593 or write to the Clinical Director, National Cancer Institute, Building 10, Room 12N214, Bethesda, MD 20892.

How will I know if I have been accepted as a patient at the Clinical Center?

If the scientists at the Center determine you are eligible, your doctor will be notified. Occasionally it may be necessary for you to be seen at the Clinical Center for a preliminary interview and study of your case. The Clinical Center provides nursing and medical care without charge for patients who are being studied in clinical research programs. However, the Center generally cannot pay transportation costs.

UNPROVEN METHODS

What You Need to Know about Unproven Treatments

- For many who want to explore approaches to self-care that would improve their quality of life, such as meditation, deep relaxation, hypnosis, imagery, a wholesome balanced vegetarian diet, psychological or spiritual support, and the traditional Chinese medicine, there are ethical and appropriately qualified practitioners available locally at moderate cost.
- If you are using an unproven method in combination with standard treatment, it is important to discuss it with your health care team to make sure that it does not interfere with your treatment and to review potential side effects.

There may be a risk, for instance, in mixing some chemo-therapy drugs with unorthodox substances.

- Usually there is little scientific evidence presented by those promoting unproven methods. Patients are encouraged to have the treatment even though there is no true evidence that it really works. There are some promoters who engage in unethical sales techniques, make misleading promises, charge high fees, and neglect prudent conventional medical supervision and care. Many times the write-ups for the unproven methods use scientific words or phrases in a misleading manner.

- Some treatments that have been tested and found useless, such as laetrile, are renamed and repackaged and continue to be sold to unsuspecting patients.

- Although some unproven methods are being prescribed by physicians, many cures are being promoted by doctors with unrecognizable degrees such as N.D. (doctor of naturopathy), Ph.N. (philosopher of naturopathy), D.A.B.B-A. (Diplomate of the American Board of Bio-Analysts), and Ms.D. (doctor of metaphysics).

- Recent changes in regulations of the U.S. Food and Drug Administration (FDA), especially the Dietary Supplement and Health Education Act of 1994, created a new category that includes vitamins, minerals, herbs, amino acids, and other "supplements" and allows products to go to market with no testing for efficacy. These products do not have to be manufactured according to any standards. Claims are permitted on packages. Although labels may not claim to cure or prevent a disease, they may detail how a supplement affects the body's structure or function as long as claims are truthful and not misleading. For example, saw palmetto, an herb, can't claim that it will cure an enlarged prostate, but it can claim to improve urinary flow or say that it is "for the prostate." Many consumers still believe that any product that appears in pill form has been reviewed for safety by the FDA. This is not true for supplements, so be aware of the products you are buying. The label does have to say that any claims have *not* been reviewed or approved by the FDA, so read the small print carefully.

• The magazine *Consumer Reports* has continuing articles on the subject of health issues. "Herbal Roulette" in the November 1995 issue details many of the herbal remedies that are unregulated and gives hints on how to protect yourself.

> It has been interesting to us that some of the patients who are most adamant about asking their doctors to prove whether or not conventional treatment works accept as fact the information given by a friend or by a clerk in a health food store. There is no question that many people are disillusioned with and fearful of many standard treatments and therefore turn to alternative or nontoxic therapies. It's easy to be lured into trying unproven methods of treatment by the promise of a cure. Our advice is to ask hard questions about the unproven methods— as many and as detailed as you do about your regular treatment or about clinical trials. Use your own good common sense. If you decide to try an alternative method, do your homework. Be a wary consumer. Remember that if it sounds too good to be true, it probably is.

What is the difference between investigational treatment and unproven methods?

Investigational treatments, also called clinical trials or experimental treatments, use specific scientific methods and standards to evaluate new therapies or procedures. Unproven methods, sometimes called alternative treatment, cannot be proven effective either because no studies exist or because whatever data are available have not been produced using the specific standards and methods required of scientific research. Although the standards being used for investigational treatment are complex and strict, they are put in place for the safety of the public and to make sure that any new treatment offered to patients actually works.

What is the Office of Alternative Medicine at the National Institutes of Health?

The primary interest of this office, established in 1992, is to investigate alternative treatments even if the way those treatments work is not fully understood. It has begun to fund research in areas such as acupuncture, biofeedback, hypnosis, music therapy, massage therapy, yoga, and prayer as they relate to many different diseases including cancer. It gives an opportunity to demonstrate scientific validity to those who are practicing alternative medicine. The Office of Alternative Medicine has funded eight specialty research centers for ongoing alternative medicine research. The University of Texas Health Science Center in Houston was granted the award for research in cancer.

What do I need to be aware of when looking at unproven treatments?

We feel that it is important for you to be an informed consumer in assessing any cures reported in the popular press. Ask the hard questions about the unproven methods being offered, and do your own research into what is promising. Use your own common sense and sound judgment.

Why are doctors often opposed to unproven treatments?

Most doctors feel that there are risks to patients using an unproven method instead of a conventional, proven treatment. The most substantial risk is the delay in getting a treatment that could offer a cure. Many standard treatments are highly successful, especially in curing cancers that are found early. If you use an unproven treatment first and then try the standard treatment after the unproven one does not work, your cancer may be in an advanced stage and be more difficult to cure.

QUESTIONS TO ASK BEFORE USING UNPROVEN METHODS

- Why do I want to use this kind of treatment?
- What do I think it will accomplish?
- What evidence is there that the unproven method will work? How has it been evaluated?
- Has it been written up in a scientific journal? Why not?
- Do the practitioners of the method claim that the medical community is trying to keep their cure from the public?

- Does the treatment have a "secret formula" that only a small group of practitioners know about?
- Has the treatment been evaluated by an independent group of researchers?
- How long has the establishment been in operation? Is it certified by any authoritative body?
- What are the qualifications of the people who will be treating me? Have they graduated from accredited schools?
- Does it sound too good to be true?
- Have I discussed the treatment with my doctor?
- Will the doctor continue to care for me if I am using this treatment?
- Can I continue my regular treatments and try the unproven method at the same time?
- Is there some kind of investigational or experimental treatment that would give the same or better results?
- Is the treatment being tested by the Office of Alternative Medicine?
- What costs will be associated with the unproven method?
- How do these costs compare with conventional treatment?
- Will my health insurance reimburse me for these costs?

CARNIVORA CURE

What is the carnivora cure?

This is a treatment that, as far as we are able to verify, is available through Dr. Helmut Keller of the Chronic Disease Control and Treatment Center, Bad Steben, Germany. It is used in conjunction with full-body hyperthermia along with a regimen of vitamins and minerals. Dr. Keller discovered the cancer-killing properties of the Venus's-flytrap plant when he was working on tumorigenesis in the animal laboratories of Boston University. Hydroplumbagin-4-O-beta-glucopyranoside, or plumbagin, a main component of carnivora, was isolated in 1988.

As we were about to go to press, we received this letter from a dear friend who had been given a diagnosis of prostate cancer about six months ago and was undecided about what path to take. While doing his research, he was put on hormone therapy. His research led him down many paths, and his conclusions were unconventional and a bit of a surprise.

"I have made a decision to go with a combination of traditional and alternative medicine for my prostate cancer. With an encouraging blood immunology report just received and a PSA reading of 0.008 down from 7.1 originally, thanks to the hormonal treatment, I have decided to act. My decision flows from a six-month study and from my relationship with my urologist, a lot of consultation and more than a little praying.

"Early on I began attending support meetings and saw what successful men were doing to take charge of their cancer. They were establishing partnerships with their doctors and were sharing in their own recovery program as active participants and decision makers. I will go to be treated in Bad Steben, Germany, by Dr. Helmut Keller and his medical group for a period of approximately one month to six weeks. I will have hyperthermia and carnivora, minerals, and other medications for strengthening my immune system.

"My decision was not an easy call, but I feel that the value of one of the established traditional therapies to eradicate the tumor and one of the complementary or alternative therapies to rebuild the immune system is right for me."

MACROBIOTIC DIET

What is the macrobiotic diet?

The macrobiotic diet, also known as the Zen macrobiotic diet, consists mainly of cereal products, such as rice. Individuals following the diet must not eat any sugar, meat, or animal products and must restrict their intake of fluids. There are many variations of the macrobiotic diet. The principle of all of the diets is that liquids, usually in the form of miso or tamari broth, be used only sparingly. Meats (including poultry), dairy products, tropical or semitropical fruits and juices, sugar, honey, and anything artificial are to be avoided. The most restrictive of these diets, not usually followed today, uses only cereals, mostly in the form of brown rice. Those who recommend the diet for cancer patients believe that cancer is a toxic blood condition that has developed because of poor eating habits.

METABOLIC THERAPY

What is metabolic therapy?

Metabolic therapy consists of flushing out the body's toxins and supplying a well-balanced diet along with various vitamins and enzymes. The diet is vegetarian with emphasis on raw "live" foods and fresh vegetable juices. Sugar, white flour products, processed foods of any kind, coffee, and alcoholic beverages are not permitted. A number of programs fall into the metabolic therapy umbrella, including Gerson therapy, laetrile, and the Hoxsey treatment.

What is Gerson therapy?

Gerson therapy aims to rid the body of toxins and flood the cells with nutrients. The diet includes organically grown fresh vegetables and fruits, thirteen glasses of freshly squeezed juices daily, including raw liver juice, as well as linseed oil and a handful of naturally occurring mineral supplements. A coffee enema is administered several times a day to cleanse the body of toxins.

What is laetrile?

Laetrile is a product made from apricot pits that contains a chemical called amygdalin. Promoters of laetrile, which is also called vitamin B_{17}, claim that it is a harmless, effective treatment for cancer and useful in cancer prevention. However, no scientific evidence supports these claims. The National Cancer Institute tested laetrile in laboratory animals several times but found no convincing evidence that it is effective against animal cancers.

However, because of widespread public use and interest in the subject, the National Cancer Institute conducted a clinical study of laetrile with cancer patients. The conclusion of the researchers who participated in the trial was that laetrile was ineffective as a treatment for cancer and did not substantially improve symptoms of the disease in the patients studied. A detailed report of the study was published in *The New England Journal of Medicine* in January 1982 (Vol. 306, No. 4).

What is the Hoxey treatment?

This treatment consists mainly of a tonic made of herbs that is prescribed for internal cancers and a powder, salve, or clear solution for external cancers. After many legal battles, the FDA banned the sale of all Hoxey treatments in 1960. However, the treatment is still available in Mexico.

What is the Burton treatment?

Dr. Lawrence Burton offers a treatment called immunoaugmentative therapy. He originally practiced in New York (though he is, by profession, a zoologist) and because of legal difficulties is located in the Grand Bahama Islands. His treatment involves a serum made of a combination of human blood agents. The treatment materials have not been licensed for sale by the FDA and scientific evidence to confirm the anticancer properties of his products is lacking. Because Dr. Burton's research data have not been published, other scientists have not been able to evaluate his claims.

SAW PALMETTO COMPLEX (*SERENOA REPENS*)

What is *Serenoa repens*?

Serenoa repens is an extract made from the berries of the saw palmetto tree. The extract works by blocking the production of 5-alpha-reductase, which is known to convert testosterone to dihydrotestosterone. It also may inhibit production of 3-alpha-reductase, which is thought to play a role in prostate enlargement and keeps dihydrotestosterone from binding to the cell receptors in the prostate. Its primary use is not in treating prostate cancer but in decreasing prostate enlargement and relieving frequent and painful urination. It is available in health food stores as saw palmetto complex and Pro-Sanoa.

SHARK CARTILAGE

What is shark cartilage treatment?

Proponents of shark cartilage treatment say that an insignificant number of sharks—one out of a million or less—get cancer and that sharks seem to resist tumors naturally. Rather than bones, the skeletons of sharks are made of pure cartilage, a hard gristly material formed from proteins and complex carbohydrates and toughened by rodlike fibers. They feel that prostate, breast, cervical, central nervous system, and pancreatic cancers, because they are the most heavily vascularized cancers, will be the most likely to be affected by shark cartilage.

Are any research scientists studying shark cartilage?

Scientists discovered in 1984 that cartilage contains substances that can inhibit the development of the network of blood vessels that tumors need for nourishment. They say that the shark is not the only creature that has tissues composed of cartilage. Cartilage tissues similar in structure and composition to those of the shark skeleton are present in most of the joints of the human body and ordinarily resist invasion by tumor cells and blood cells. Scientists are working in an area called antiangiogenesis, studying how these tissue inhibitors work, and are trying to develop drugs based on these inhibitors. The value of shark cartilage has not been proven.

VACCINES

What is the Livingston treatment?

The basis of this treatment is a vaccine prepared from a culture of the patient's own bacteria given in conjunction with the tuberculosis vaccine. Use of these vaccines at the Livingston-Wheeler Clinic in San Diego, California, reflected Livingston's belief that cancer is caused by a microbe. Nutrition is an important part of the treatment, primarily a live-food vegetarian diet, with all poultry forbidden. The California Department of Health Services Cancer Advisory Council, which included nine cancer experts and five consumer representatives, conducted a review of the available information and concluded that there is no scientific basis for believing that the vaccines are safe and effective for the treatment of cancer. As a result, in 1990, the state of California ordered the clinic to stop treating cancer patients with these vaccines, which were not approved by the FDA.

chapter 15

What Can I Do about Sex, Incontinence and Other Side Effects?

Impotence and incontinence (and not always necessarily in that order) are the most feared side effects of many of the treatments for prostate cancer, so the possibilities of weakened bladder control or nonexistent erections need to be considered along with some of the other side effects of the treatments. The general side effects are discussed in this chapter. Those specific to the type of treatment, such as surgery, radiation therapy, radiation seeding, hormonal therapy, and cryosurgery, are covered in the appropriate chapters.

After treatment for prostate cancer, many men have sexual and urinary problems, but these problems can clear up over time.

SEXUAL PROBLEMS AFTER TREATMENT

Some erectile dysfunction has been found to be caused by the physical and emotional aftereffects of treatment. Most experts suggest that it is important to be patient and wait at least six months to a year to see if function will return. Meanwhile, you may find it helpful to discuss your sexual concerns with your physician, an oncology clinical nurse specialist, a sex therapist, or sex counselor. Although no man **wants** to use a device to have sex, when faced with the choice of not being able to enjoy sex or using "something" to facilitate erections, most men are willing to at least consider trying one of a variety of possibilities available.

And by all means, express your concerns and feelings about your sexual problems with your partner. Open, honest communications are a must.

Why is it that since I've had cancer I have little or no sex drive?

This is a normal reaction to your treatments but will probably change as stress decreases. However, there is great need for physical contact, though not necessarily for sexual intercourse. Partners should be aware that the special warmth of a loving touch conveys feelings in a very direct way. You need to tell your partner how important it is for you to be touched even if you do not want to have intercourse. Try not to make your partner guess your feelings.

Why do I feel so angry about my cancer affecting my sexual relationship?

Because there is a close connection between anger and sexual feelings, problems in relationships often result from treatment for prostate cancer. Though the way anger is expressed may be different for each partner and each couple, the feelings often exist and are sometimes repressed. An important part of the healing process is to discuss these feelings openly. Once the anger has been confronted and understood, steps can be taken toward accepting it and other emotions triggered by a cancer diagnosis.

Is it possible that my partner thinks my cancer could be contagious?

If you suspect this, you need to talk with your partner about this fear. Bring the question up and try to get your partner to talk about it. Understandably, there is a great deal of anxiety about sexual transmission of disease due largely to herpes and AIDS. However, it is important for both partners to understand that cancer is **not** contagious. It is an internal process that affects the cells of the body, causing them to multiply in an uncontrolled fashion. There is absolutely no evidence to suggest that having intercourse with someone who has cancer can in any way spread the cancer to the other person. Nor will your cancer spread or recur as a result of having sexual intercourse.

If treatment makes me impotent, is there any way that I can regain sexual functioning?

If the nerves were not removed during surgery, sexual function may return, though it may take a considerable period of time, often as long as a year to several years, before it returns to normal. For those whose function will not return, there are both surgical and nonsurgical alternatives.

Why do I still have problems having an erection even though the doctor says my prostate surgery or radiation therapy was successful ?

There are many reasons why you may not be able to have an erection. It happens to every man at times—even to those who don't have cancer. Worry about cancer, depression, anxiety, being tired, trying too hard, stress, alcohol—all can result in erection problems. Any sign of an erection gives you proof that your body is cooperating, but the psyche is so sensitive that it may take quite a long time for you to feel certain enough of your performance for you to resume normal intercourse. A number of men report that they had their first orgasm after cancer treatment while asleep, during a sexual dream. If you have such an experience, it is proof that you can achieve erection, because sleep erections are not affected by psychological factors. Perhaps this is a good time for you to experiment with other pleasuring techniques. If the doctor says there is no physical reason for the problem, perhaps the cause is psychological due to pressure you feel about getting an erection. The pace of sexual adjustment after treatment often depends upon your feelings about yourself. A frank discussion with your doctor or with a sex therapist may help you gain a better understanding of the problem.

What does a sex therapist do?

A sex therapist usually wants to hear from both partners about problems and how each partner views them. Just bringing problems into the open and discussing them with a professional can be helpful.

How do I find a good sex therapist?

If your physician or other health professional cannot make a referral to a sex therapist familiar with cancer-related problems, you can get in touch with trained professionals who belong to the American Association of Sex Educators, Counselors and Therapists or the National Association of Oncology Social Workers (see Chapter 16). You may also locate members of these organizations by looking in the Yellow Pages under Marriage and Family Counseling or by consulting the American Cancer Society, Cancer Information Service, local Family Service, or United Way agencies. Before making an appointment, you may want to ask whether the therapist has had training and experience in dealing with sexual problems relating to cancer.

Should I include my partner in my decisions about how to deal with my erection problems?

Your partner is the other half of this equation, and it is important to include your partner in any decisions you make. Of course, the final decisions are yours. But you should be sure you know how your partner feels about the decisions you are making. Many men assume that their partners are first and foremost interested in having sex—and of course they are. But being practical, most would opt for having their partners live longer at the expense of sacrificing some sexual satisfaction. Most are more interested in intimacy than operative technique. Share your feelings. Talk about your fears and concerns. Discuss how changes will affect your sexual relationship and how you can both find satisfaction.

Make 2 copies of this checklist—one for you and one for your partner—and compare them when completed.

PUTTING YOUR RELATIONSHIP INTO PERSPECTIVE

	TRUE OR FALSE	DON'T WANT TO DISCUSS	DOES NOT APPLY
I want to share intimacy but am not ready for sexual intercourse.			
My partner doesn't seem interested in sex.			
I don't seem to get sexually aroused.			
I'm afraid it will hurt.			
I'm not interested in sex anymore.			
I purposely avoid sex.			
Sex is unsatisfying for me.			
I feel ashamed of not being able to have an erection.			
I feel like a failure and inadequate so it's better not even to try.			
I wish we could be more open and frank.			
I get excited but don't reach a climax.			

I hesitate about having sex because I feel it's unfair to my partner if I can't have an erection.			
I feel guilty at leaving my partner unsatisfied.			
There is no replacement for the kind of intimacy you have from real sexual intercourse.			
I don't need to have the real act of intercourse to show my expressions of love.			
I'm getting too old to enjoy sex.			
I can't seem to get an erection/climax, so I avoid sex.			
My partner doesn't want to try anything different.			
My illness has changed the way I see myself as a person.			
I'm not sure whether my partner is avoiding me, doesn't feel up to it, or just isn't interested.			
I think it's time we faced the fact that we cannot have intercourse and should discuss and try other means of physical interaction.			
I would be happy if my partner would talk with me honestly about how she/he feels about our sexual relationship.			

(continued)

PUTTING YOUR RELATIONSHIP INTO PERSPECTIVE (cont.)

	TRUE OR FALSE	DON'T WANT TO DISCUSS	DOES NOT APPLY
I find that dry ejaculation detracts from my sexual pleasure.			
I still think it's too early to decide whether erections will return.			
I'm willing to keep trying and experimenting with what works for us.			
I am afraid of catching cancer.			
I think that because I can't have intercourse I should leave my partner.			
I hate the idea of using a device to have sex.			
I think my partner is unfair to want sex when I'm having problems.			
I think it's inappropriate to be thinking about sex in the midst of a life-threatening illness.			

Statement				
I'm ready to give up the sexual factor in our relationship, but I'd like to talk about it.				
I'm satisfied with pleasurable alternatives to actual intercourse.				
I find self-stimulation is a good sexual outlet for me.				
I think we should try the injectable drug for erections.				
I think we should look into using the vacuum pump.				
I think a surgical implant pump sounds like a good solution.				
I'd be willing to try some different ways of making love.				
Sex is still good even though we have problems.				
I'm willing to see a sex counselor to discuss our problems.				
I'd like to regain the intimacy that is a fundamental aspect of our love even if we can't have sex the way we used to.				
Our love has grown deeper even with our problems.				

How can I help my partner to start talking about sexual feelings?

It is often difficult to discuss intimate feelings. Yet it can be dangerous to second-guess what your partner is thinking. The questionnaire on the previous pages was designed so that each partner could fill it out separately. Make a second copy for your partner. You can then compare notes and use what you learn about each other to gain greater understanding. This is not a test. There are no passing or failing scores. The statements merely highlight what is happening in your sexual life and may help you understand each other better.

After you have discussed your checklists together, you may want to talk about the following questions:

- How satisfied are you with the quality of closeness you share?
- How important is sexual intercourse to you as an expression of intimacy?
- How important are other means of physical interaction to you?
- What makes you feel most loved and appreciated?
- What was one recent encounter that made you feel close?
- What keeps you from becoming closer?
- What would make you happier?
- What does your partner think makes you happiest in your physical relationship?
- Are you interested in scheduling an appointment with a sex therapist?

Is there a diagnostic workup that can be done to determine whether or not the erection problems are permanent?

A diagnostic workup can be done to determine whether the problem is organic or psychological. This is usually done with a device that monitors whether or not erections occur during sleep. Normally, erections occur several times a night during sleep. When there are true organic problems, erections do not occur during sleep.

What methods are used by men with impotence from surgery or radiation to have intercourse?

There are a number of surgical and nonsurgical approaches now available including injectable drugs, vacuum devices, and penile implants. In addition, testing is underway with drugs that can be inserted into the penis with a plastic tube instead of a needle. This device is expected to be on the market in 1997. In the early stages of testing by Pfizer is the ultimate method: a simple pill that would deliver an enzyme that promotes erections. The pill, however, is not presently available and is not expected to be marketed until 1998.

What injectable drugs are available to help produce erections?

Highly effective drugs such as alprostadil (Caverject), papaverine, phentolamine, and prostaglandin E_1, used alone or in combination, produce erections in many men when injected with a very fine needle into the side of the penis. Although it sounds painful, this usually painless injection is reported to be effective in 75 to 90 percent of men. Frequent use can cause a buildup of scar tissue at the injection site. Cost of injectable drugs can run from $10 to $30 per use and is not covered by many insurance companies or by Medicare.

How do the impotence drug injections work?

The newest drug, alprostadil (Caverject), is a synthetic version of a naturally occurring form of prostaglandin E_1, which is found in human tissues and fluids and plays a role in erection by widening blood vessels. The drug is injected into the penis shortly before intercourse. It relaxes and widens the muscles in the arteries that supply blood to the penis. The increased blood flow compresses the veins against a rigid fibrous sheath. It usually induces an erection within 5 to 20 minutes. Possible side effects include mild to moderate pain at the injection site and scarring of penile tissue. A few men may have an abnormally prolonged erection. If the erection lasts more than a few hours, you need to go to the emergency room for an injection to reverse the effect of the drug.

Who gives the injection?

Usually the first injection is given by the doctor in the office, so that the dose can be adjusted as needed. You will be shown how to prepare the medication, get the correct dosage, and inject the needle. Your partner may wish to learn the technique and incorporate it as part of your sexual ritual. Most men are surprised at how easy and painless it is to use this method to encourage erections.

How do vacuum erection devices work?

There are several types of external, noninvasive vacuum devices that produce an erection. One such device is worn like a condom but is made of a semirigid material. The sheath is put on, and a vacuum is applied to draw the penis out to fill it. The device is left in place for intercourse. Another device requires putting the penis in a vacuum that draws blood into the organ. When an adequate erection has been produced, it can be maintained by placing a soft rubber ring around the base of the penis, which helps maintain the erection for about 30 minutes. These devices work, in most cases, whether or not nerves have been preserved, because they do not depend on the body to produce the erection. The vacuum forces the blood to flow into the penis. Two companies that make such devices are Osbon Medical Systems of Augusta, Georgia (1-706-821-6850), which makes ErecAid, and Mission Pharmacal Company of San Antonio, Texas, maker of the VED pump (1-800-531-3333). The cost is about $400 and may be covered by Medicare or insurance.

Are there disadvantages to using the vacuum erection device?

One disadvantage sometimes mentioned is the loss of spontaneity involved in making preparations since three to five minutes are required to produce an erection. However, some couples use the device as part of the foreplay ritual and find that this helps to turn the disadvantage into a plus. In addition, because the rigidity of a normal erection depends on the engorgement of internal tissue and only the part of the penile shaft beyond the constricting ring is engorged, the result may be a less firm erection. (Note: Many companies offer a money-back guarantee, so before purchasing, it is wise to ask if a full refund is possible if necessary.)

Are there side effects to using the vacuum erection device?

Reported possible side effects are extremely minor: a reddish rash on the penis and bruising if the vacuum pressure is maintained for too long.

How do surgically implanted devices work?

There are a number of different prosthetic designs that can help a man achieve a controlled erection. Some are simple malleable, semirigid rods that are implanted inside the penis. Newer types of inflatable penile prostheses operate hydraulically to make the penis hard or soft. A plastic reservoir about the size of a tangerine is implanted inside the body beneath muscles near the bladder. The implanted reservoir serves as a permanent storehouse for water. The reservoir is connected by two thin plastic tubes to a hydraulic pump planted in the scrotal sac, which in turn is attached to two hollow cylinders, much like balloons, that are implanted in the penis. To achieve an erection, the small pump is gently squeezed. This releases the salt water in the reservoir, which flows down into the cylinders and creates the erection. The fluid returns to the reservoir when a release valve implanted inside the scrotum is pressed. Another type involves a series of interlocking plastic blocks that can be inflated or deflated by a spring-loaded cable that passes through them.

What kind of doctor specializes in these implants?

Most urologists can implant these devices. Before arranging for an implant, it might be wise to determine how successful your urologist has been with this surgery. It might be helpful, also, to get the names of some of his patients who have had the surgery so that you can discuss their experience.

Does the body sometimes reject these implants?

Prophylactic antibiotics are used, and most times the implants are successful. Only about one percent of implants is rejected or creates infections. In those cases, the prosthesis is removed and the infection is treated. Many times the prosthesis can be reimplanted.

How long does penile implant surgery take?

Implant surgery takes from about 30 minutes to two hours. Many patients spend two to five days recuperating in the hospital. Full recovery requires four to six weeks. The usual complications of surgery are possible. Infection, bleeding, and abnormal scarring do sometimes occur. On the whole, complication rates are low. Although no mechanical device is a perfect replacement, most men who have had the surgery say they are satisfied with the implant results. As might be expected, the cost of implants and surgery can run well into thousands of dollars. Costs are usually covered by insurance.

How does the single-dose drug plunger applicator work?

Still in the testing stage, this system, called MUSE (medicated urethral system for erection), is scheduled to be on the market in 1997. One or two drugs, alprostadil and prozosin, are inserted with a tiny plunger about the size of an eye dropper into the penis and produce an erection within 10 minutes that lasts up to an hour. It appears to work best for men who get partial erections or who can achieve erections only sporadically. The device is being developed by Vivus, Inc., Menlo Park, California.

Are there any natural oral medications that can help with erections?

Those involved in the natural medicine field cite yohimbine, a drug extracted from the bark of the yohimbine tree, as having properties that raises the libido. It is often used with the antidepressant trazodone. It is said to improve erections in about a third of users, especially those with psychologically caused impotence. Its biological activity has not been proven, and it is considered by some to be a placebo.

Is there an organization that deals with impotence problems?

The Impotence Institute of America, Inc., provides information on impotence and its treatment. (See Chapter 16.)

URINARY PROBLEMS

Urinary problems are an unwanted side effect for many men who have prostate cancer. Dealing with these problems is very difficult for most men, and an understanding of the problem is important. If you become incontinent after treatment, there are several ways of dealing with the problem.

Is incontinence sometimes temporary?

In many cases, incontinence is temporary and improves over time. It may be helped with corrective exercises, known as Kegel exercises, or through behavior modification—scheduling of bathroom visits to train the bladder to hold urine longer. These techniques can hasten the recovery from temporary incontinence after surgery. Sometimes, however, the incontinence persists and may become a permanent condition.

How are Kegel exercises done?

Kegel exercises are designed to strengthen perineal muscles.

- Empty your bladder. Try to relax completely.
- Tense your muscles by pressing your buttocks together. Hold this position and count to 10.
- Now relax and count to 10.
- Do this exercise for 10 minutes each time, three times a day. At the beginning, you may not be able to hold the position for the count of 10 or you may tire before you have completed the entire set. If so, stop exercising and go back to it later, gradually increasing the number and length of each set.

Are there other suggestions that help to improve incontinence?

- When starting to void, shut off the stream for a few seconds, then start voiding again. Do this exercise each time you urinate to improve urinary control.
- Remember to urinate as soon as you feel the need. Do not wait.
- It may take several weeks or months of daily exercise before you notice a difference.

What are some practical ways of dealing with incontinence after a prostatectomy?

Many men find that incontinence can be managed with the use of incontinence pads, available at most drugstores, that can be slipped into undershorts or shorts with additional padding to catch any dribbles. There are also external collection devices made of rubber, similar to a condom. These are pulled over the penis and held in place by a band around the waist. A tube for drainage is connected to the collection bag, which is secured to the leg by a band. A penile clamp can be used to control the flow of urine. You must be careful not to apply too much pressure, because the clamp might restrict blood flow through the penis. One support group told us about a less sophisticated but very practical method. They use small Baggies filled with either a pad or tissues and secured with a twistie wire.

How does the doctor decide what is causing my long-term incontinence?

There are several major causes of incontinence in men who have been treated for prostate cancer: damage to the bladder neck, the sphincter muscles, or other muscles around the prostate gland. The doctor will do a physical examination and take a detailed history of your problem. It is helpful if you keep a diary that tracks how often you urinate, when you leak, what activities (such as exercise, walking, and sneezing) you are doing when you leak, and how many pads you use. This will help the doctor diagnose your specific problem. You may also have a urodynamic test to reproduce your specific symptoms, a cystoscopy (bladder exam), or an ultrasound exam.

What are the most common treatments for long-term incontinence?

Doctors often suggest behavioral techniques or prescribe drugs. Learning behavior modification techniques is time-consuming, usually requiring one one-hour session per week for 8 to 12 weeks. Although behavior modification is effective in more than 50 percent of patients, it may not be covered by insurance. The cost varies from $500 to several thousand dollars.

What drugs are used for long-term incontinence?

Several drugs, including oxybutynin, imipramine, and hyoscyamine, are used to treat severe incontinence. These drugs relax bladder muscles and inhibit spasms. You may have some side effects, such as dry mouth and constipation. The cost is about $50 a month.

Is electrical stimulation used to treat incontinence?

Electrical stimulation is being studied. It includes a probe that delivers electrical stimulation for a few seconds several times every day for several weeks. Early results show promise for this treatment.

What do collagen implants do for incontinence?

To prevent leakage, collegen is injected into the body of the urethra to reinforce the sphincter muscle by adding tissue. (The collagen is made from a protein extract of connective tissue from cows and purified for human use.) A skin test is done beforehand to determine that you are not allergic to the substance. Doctors who perform this procedure are required by the Food and Drug Administration to receive special training. The collagen is injected though a flexible needle into the tissue at the bladder neck. Collagen injections are performed with either local or general anesthetia. The treatment can be repeated; a number of treatments is usually required to achieve results. Because several syringes of collagen, costing several hundred dollars each, are usually used for each treatment, the cost for this treatment usually is several thousand dollars.

Can incontinence be treated with surgery?

It depends on your problem and what damage has been done by past surgery. One operation strengthens the ring of muscle at the opening of your bladder, called the sphincter. Be sure, before you have anything done, that you understand the extent of the operation, the expected results, how many such operations your doctor has performed and how successful they have been, the side effects of the operation and what other treatment might be used instead of surgery. You might also ask to talk to a patient who has had a similar operation so that you can understand what to expect from a patient's point of view.

Are there implanted devices for long-term urinary problems?

There are devices similar to the penile implants that are sometimes used to solve the problems of urine control. A reservoir is implanted, which is controlled by a small pump implanted in the scrotum. A cuff is implanted around the urethra. When the cuff relaxes as the control pump is squeezed, the urine gathered in the bladder is released. The cuff closes on its own in about two minutes. The system automatically repressurizes until the body signals the need to urinate again. Data show that these implants are effective in about 80 percent of patients, but they require major surgery.

Does diet play a part in incontinence?

Diet can lead to incontinence, because obesity puts pressure on the bladder, as does lack of exercise. Try to avoid alcohol and caffeine in coffee, tea, and soft drinks. Don't limit your intake of fluids, thinking this will help. Too little liquid can increase your incontinence problem and result in constipation. It is, however, a good idea to limit your fluid intake at night to one or two cups after your evening meal.

Can medications cause incontinence?

Drugs that you may be taking for other medical problems may play a role in incontinence. High blood pressure drugs (beta-blockers) can weaken the sphincter muscle. Antihistamines and sleeping pills may also be problematic.

Are there any organizations that deal specifically with incontinence?

There are two: Help for Incontinent People, which can provide information and referrals, and the Simon Foundation for Continence, which gives information on the management and treatment of incontinence (see Chapter 16).

OTHER SIDE EFFECTS

Is blood in my urine or semen cause for alarm?

It is frightening to discover blood in the urine or semen, and the presence of blood can be an indication of serious problems. However, many times when blood is seen in the urine, it may be the result of broken blood vessels on the surface of the prostate, prostate or bladder infections, bladder tumors, or kidney stones. Blood in the semen may be caused by an inflammation or irritation of the prostate or seminal vesicles. Sometimes after radiation, blood appears in the urine—even a year or more after treatment. This can be caused by radiation damage, which may have weakened tissue and blood vessels in the bladder and prostate. It is important to have your urologist evaluate the problem so that the cause can be determined.

What is retrograde or dry ejaculation?

In retrograde ejaculation, the semen goes backward into the bladder rather than through the urethra and out the penis. This side effect can result from several prostate treatments. Some men complain that this changes the pleasurable sensation of orgasm. For most men, however, the only reminder of this change is the slightly cloudy urine seen after intercourse. For men who want to father children, it is possible to isolate the semen from the urine voided after ejaculation. The recovered semen can be used for artificial insemination. Of course, for men who have had a radical prostatectomy, this would not be possible since there is no ejaculate.

How are symptoms of bone metastases caused by prostate cancer treated?

If prostate cancer spreads to the lymph nodes and to the blood-producing tissues of the bone marrow, feelings of weakness and fatigue may result. Sometimes weight-bearing bones will fracture. There are a number of avenues that can be followed to control severe pain. Hormone therapy is usually the mainstay of treatment. If the bone metastasis is confined to one area, external beam radiation may be used. Strontium-89 (Metastron) is a radioactive substance that is sometimes injected into the veins to kill cancer cells in the bone. One injection can give relief up to six months and can be repeated.

What can be done about bladder irritation?

Bladder irritation, which can cause burning during urination or the sense of urgency to urinate, can be a very annoying side effect. Sometimes your doctor can prescribe medications to relax the bladder and make it less irritable.

What should I do if my urinary stream slows down and I have trouble urinating?

This can sometimes happen during the first three months after prostate surgery. If it does, you should notify your doctor. It can be treated by passing a dilating instrument through the urethra or be corrected with minor surgery. Once this complication is treated, it usually does not persist or recur.

What kind of rectal problems can result from prostate cancer treatment?

Pain, frequent bowel movements, bleeding, chronic burning, and rectal discharge sometimes occur. Your doctor may be able to prescribe medications to help ease these side effects.

What can be done about diarrhea?

Avoid foods that give you gas, cause cramps, and irritate your
bowels, such as cereals high in fiber, raw vegetables, fruits, coffee,
and milk products. Foods rich in minerals such as bananas, potatoes, and apricots can help replace those lost because of diarrhea. Rice, bananas, applesauce, dry toast, mashed potatoes, and
crackers are helpful for controlling diarrhea.

What is lymphedema?

Lymphedema is an accumulation of lymph fluid that may cause
swelling in the legs and genitals following the removal of lymph
nodes. It is a rare but possible side effect of surgery and radiation
treatment. Lymphedema can occur soon after treatment or even
as many as 15 years later. When chronic lymphedema develops,
it is a lifelong condition that requires constant monitoring and
therapy. Positioning, massage, exercise, special garments, and
pumps are all used in treating lymphedema (see Chapters 8 and
9).

Are there any other side effects of treatment?

See Chapters 8 through 13 for information on possible side effects
of specific treatments.

SUPPORT GROUPS

How do I find appropriate support groups?

There are two general kinds of support groups available: support
groups led by health professionals and self-help groups that are
run by people who have prostate cancer. Some groups offer support, some education; some are for patients alone, some for family
members, and some for both. There are groups that include people with different kinds of cancer and some that are made up
only of men with prostate cancer. Some are less traditional and
focus on alternative techniques such as visualization, relaxation,
and meditation. All offer encouragement, information, strategies
for coping, and a wonderful place to form friendships with others
who understand your problems. The American Cancer Society offices in local communities often have a variety of support groups.

Their *I Can Cope* program addresses the educational and psychological needs of people with cancer and their families. A series of eight classes are set up to discuss cancer, how to cope with daily health problems, how to express feelings, living with limitations, and available local resources. You can check with your doctor, the social services department of your hospital, the Cancer Information Service, or the American Cancer Society in your area for more information about available groups.

What is PAACT?

The organization Patient Advocates for Advanced Cancer Treatments (PAACT) is a clearinghouse for information on prostate cancer treatments. Their focus is on nonsurgical treatments—primarily combination hormone therapy, cryotherapy, and suramin. Membership includes a subscription to *The Cancer Communication Newsletter.*

Are there support groups especially for men with prostate cancer?

Groups for men with prostate cancer are springing up all over the country. They offer newly diagnosed patients and those who have undergone treatment a chance to get information about different treatment options, prognosis, and posttreatment follow-up in a relaxed atmosphere. Us Too and Man to Man are two support groups for prostate cancer patients with chapters around the country. Many local hospitals also have support groups specifically for men with prostate cancer. There are special support groups for partners and families. For information about support groups in your area, you can contact the Cancer Information Service, the American Cancer Society, the American Urological Association or the Prostate Cancer Support Network (see Chapter 16). There are also groups that have formed on the Internet (see Chapter 16).

chapter 16

Where to Get Help

Listings in this chapter are focused on organizations that operate on a national level. There are also many local or regional organizations that are too numerous to mention. This listing is just a starting point for your information search. The listings in this chapter are up-to-date at the time of publication. When you contact them, you may find some of your inquiries routed to different offices, organizations, and individuals.

QUICK REFERENCE FOR ESSENTIAL NUMBERS

CANCER INFORMATION SERVICE
1-800-4-CANCER
1-800-422-6237

AMERICAN CANCER SOCIETY
1-800-ACS-2345

CANCERFAX
301-402-5874

AMERICAN BOARD OF MEDICAL SPECIALTIES
1-800-776-CERT

PROSTATE CANCER GENETIC RESEARCH STUDY
1-800-777-3035

CANCER INFORMATION SERVICE

> **CALL**
> **1-800-4-CANCER**
> **(1-800-422-6237)**
> World Wide Web: http://wwwicic.nci.nih.gov/
>
> The Cancer Information Service covers the entire United States. Based on the area code from which you are dialing, you will be connected to the regional center that covers your area. All offices are open from 9:00 A.M. to 4:30 P.M.

The Cancer Information Service, a program of the National Cancer Institute, has a nationwide toll-free telephone service for cancer patients and their families, the public, and health care professionals. The Cancer Information Service information specialists can provide rapid access to the latest information on cancer and local resources. The staffs, located in regional offices across the country, have extensive training in providing up-to-date and understandable information. They can:

- Explain diagnostic procedures.
- Help you decide what questions to ask the doctor.
- Tell you about standard treatments, using PDQ, a computerized database of the National Cancer Institute.
- Conduct a computer search to give you information on where investigational treatment is being done.
- Help you explore referrals and medical facilities.
- Send free printed material.
- Discuss rehabilitation assistance and home-care assistance programs.
- Help you find financial aid or emotional counseling services.
- Discuss prevention.
- Give you information on the causes of cancer.
- Answer questions in English and Spanish.
- Help you to get answers to any questions you might have.

CancerNet
National Cancer Institute
Bethesda, MD 20892
http://wwwicic.nci.nih.gov/
A quick and easy way to get, via your computer, cancer information from the National Cancer Institute, it can be accessed through a number of different networks including Internet's Wide Wide Web and BITNET. There is no charge for the service except for your local computer charges for the use of e-mail. You can obtain information statements from the National Cancer Institute's PDQ system as well as patient publications, information about the Cancer Information Service, the National Cancer Institute's programs, and other resources. (Other Internet sources are discussed later in this chapter.)

CancerFax
National Cancer Institute
Bethesda, MD 20892
301-402-5874
301-402-7403 (for technical assistance)
This is a quick and easy way to obtain cancer information from the National Cancer Institute by calling the CancerFax computer from your fax machine. It operates 24 hours a day, seven days a week, with no charge other than a telephone call from your fax machine to the CancerFax computer in Bethesda, Maryland. You can request information statements in English or Spanish from the National Cancer Institute's PDQ system as well as fact sheets on various cancer topics from the National Cancer Institute's Office of Cancer Communications.

AMERICAN CANCER SOCIETY

American Cancer Society
Call 1-800-ACS-2345
(1-800-227-2345)
World Wide Web: http://www.cancer.org/

In most areas of the country, this number is answered at the state office of the American Cancer Society. To reach your local unit, look in the white pages of the telephone book under American Cancer Society. Ask for the person in charge of patient services.

The American Cancer Society is the nationwide, community-based, voluntary health organization. It is composed of 57 chartered divisions and nearly 3,000 local units. The national society administers programs of research, medical grants, and clinical fellowships and is charged with carrying out public and professional education at the national level. The divisions are in all states in addition to six metropolitan areas, the District of Columbia, and Puerto Rico.

The units of the American Cancer Society conduct basic service programs, including:

- Support groups such as Man to Man and Us, Too.
- Answering many questions by telephone and offering printed material on cancer free of charge.
- Information and counseling for the cancer patient and the patient's family.
- Information and guidance concerning American Cancer Society services, community health services, and other resources, such as providing transportation to and from a doctor's office, clinic, or hospital for treatment.
- Some also provide home health care, blood programs, and employment and social-work assistance.

National Office

1599 Clifton Road N.E.
Atlanta, GA 30329
1-800-ACS-2345

Division Offices

Alabama

504 Brookwood Boulevard
!Homewood, AL 35209
205-879-2242

Alaska

1057 West Fireweed Lane
Anchorage, AK 99503
907-277-8696

Arizona

2929 East Thomas Road
Phoenix, AZ 85016
602-224-0524

Arkansas

901 North University
Little Rock, AR 72203
501-664-3480

California

1710 Webster Street
Oakland, CA 96412
510-893-7900

Colorado

2255 South Oneida
Denver, CO 80224
303-758-2030

Connecticut

Barnes Park South
14 Village Lane
Wallingford, CT 06492
203-265-7161

Delaware

92 Read's Way
Suite 205
New Castle, DE 19720
302-324-4227

District of Columbia

1875 Connecticut Avenue,
  N.W.
Suite 730
Washington, DC 20009
202-483-2600

Florida

3709 West Jetton Avenue
Tampa, FL 33629-5146
813-253-0541

Georgia

2200 Lake Boulevard
Atlanta, GA 30319
404-816-7800

Hawaii Pacific

Community Services Center
 Building
200 North Vineyard Boulevard
Suite 100A
Honolulu, HI 96817
808-531-1662

Idaho

2676 Vista Avenue
Boise, ID 83705-0386
208-343-4609

Illinois

77 East Monroe
Chicago, IL 60603-5795
312-641-6150

Indiana

8730 Commerce Park Place
Indianapolis, IN 46268
317-872-4432

Iowa

8364 Hickman Road
Des Moines, IA 50325
515-253-0147

Kansas

1315 S.W. Arrowhead Road
Topeka, KS 66604
913-273-4114

Kentucky

701 West Muhammad Ali
 Boulevard
Louisville, KY 40201-1807
502-584-6782

Louisiana

2200 Veteran's Memorial
 Boulevard
Kenner, LA 70062
504-469-0021

Maine

52 Federal Street
Brunswick, ME 04011
207-729-3339

Maryland

8219 Town Center Drive
Baltimore, MD 21236-0026
410-931-6850

Massachusetts

30 Speen Street
Framingham, MA 01701-9376
508-270-4600

Michigan

1205 East Saginaw Street
Lansing, MI 48906
517-371-2920

Minnesota

3316 West 66th Street
Minneapolis, MN 55435
612-925-2772

Mississippi

1380 Livingston Lane
Lakeover Office Park
Jackson, MI 39213
601-362-8874

Missouri

3322 American Avenue
Jefferson City, MO 65102
314-893-4800

Montana

17 North 26th Street
Billings, MT 59101
406-252-7111

Nebraska

8502 West Center Road
Omaha, NE 68124-5255
402-393-5800

Nevada

1325 East Harmon
Las Vegas, NV 89119
702-798-6857

New Hampshire

360 Route 101, Unit 501
Bedford, NH 03110-5032
603-472-8899

New Jersey

2600 US Highway 1
North Brunswick, NJ 08902-
    0803
908-297-8000

New Mexico

5800 Lomas Boulevard, NE
Albuquerque, NM 87110
505-260-2105

New York State

6725 Lyons Street
East Syracuse, NY 13057
315-437-7025

LONG ISLAND

75 Davids Drive
Hauppauge, NY 11788
516-436-7070

NEW YORK CITY

19 West 56th Street
New York, NY 10019
212-586-8700

QUEENS

112-25 Queens Boulevard
Forest Hills, NY 11375
718-263-2224

WESTCHESTER

2 Lyon Place
White Plains, NY 10601
914-949-4800

North Carolina

11 South Boylan Avenue
Raleigh, NC 27603
919-834-8463

North Dakota

123 Roberts Street
Fargo, ND 58102
701-232-1385

Ohio

5555 Frantz Road
Dublin, OH 43017
614-889-9565

Oklahoma

4323 63rd, Suite 110
Oklahoma City, OK 73116
405-843-9888

Oregon

0330 S.W. Curry
Portland, OR 97201
503-295-6422

Pennsylvania

Route 422 & Sipe Avenue
Hershey, PA 17033-0897
717-533-6144

PHILADELPHIA

1422 Chestnut Street
Philadelphia, PA 19102
215-665-2900

Puerto Rico

Calle Alverio No. 577
Esquina Sargento Medina
Hato Rey, PR 00918
809-764-2295

Rhode Island

400 Main Street
Pawtucket, RI 02860
401-722-8480

South Carolina

128 Stonemark Lane
Columbia, SC 29210-3855
803-750-1693

South Dakota

4101 Carnegie Place
Sioux Falls, SD 57106-2322
605-361-8277

Tennessee

1315 Eighth Avenue, South
Nashville, TN 37203
615-255-1227

Texas

2433 Ridgepoint Drive
Austin, TX 75356
512-928-2262

Utah

941 East 3300 South
Salt Lake City, UT 84106
801-483-1500

Vermont

13 Loomis Street
Montpelier, VT 05602
802-223-2348

Virginia

4240 Park Place Court
Glen Allen, VA 23060
804-527-3700

Washington

2120 First Avenue, North
Seattle, WA 98109-1140
206-283-1152

West Virginia

2428 Kanawha Boulevard East
Charleston, WV 25311
304-344-3611

Wisconsin

N19 W24350 Riverwood Drive
Waukesha, WI 53188
414-523-5500

Wyoming

4202 Ridge Road
Cheyenne, WY 82001
307-638-3331

CANCER CENTERS AND HOSPITALS

NATIONAL CANCER INSTITUTE

National Cancer Institute
National Institutes of Health
Bethesda, MD 20892

The National Cancer Institute is the federal government's principal agency for research on cancer prevention, diagnosis, treatment, and rehabilitation and dissemination of information for the control of cancer. It is 1 of 11 research institutes and 4 divisions that form the National Institutes of Health, located in Bethesda, Maryland. As an agency of the Department of Health and Human Services, the National Cancer Institute receives annual appropriations from Congress. These funds support cancer research in the institute's Bethesda headquarters and in about 1,000 laboratories and medical centers throughout the United States. The National Cancer Institute also conducts research and treats a limited number of patients in specific research studies at the National Institutes of Health Clinical Center (see Warren Grant Magnuson Clinical Center) located in Bethesda, Maryland.

The National Cancer Institute is responsible for the Cancer Centers Program, which is made up of 55 National Cancer Institute–designated cancer centers actively engaged in multidisciplinary research efforts to reduce cancer incidence, morbidity, and mortality. Within this program there are four tiers of cancer centers:

1. Twenty-seven Comprehensive Cancer Centers, which emphasize a multidisciplinary approach to cancer research, patient care, and community outreach.
2. Seventeen Clinical Cancer Centers, which focus on clinical research.
3. One Consortium Cancer Center, which specializes in cancer prevention and control research.
4. Ten Basic Science Cancer Centers, which engage primarily in basic cancer research.

Many people choose to go to one of these major centers either for treatment or for a second opinion.

COMPREHENSIVE CANCER CENTERS

The 27 comprehensive cancer centers are designated as centers of excellence, having met specific National Cancer Institute criteria established for "comprehensiveness." It is the top designation given by the National Cancer Institute after vigorous review. The centers investigate and provide the latest scientific knowledge to doctors who are treating cancer patients. Comprehensive cancer centers have teams of experts working together on research, teaching, and patient care. They are carrying out the newest investigational treatments for cancer, using clinical trials.

Alabama

Comprehensive Cancer Center
University of Alabama at
  Birmingham
1824 Sixth Avenue South,
  Room 108
Birmingham, AL 35294-3300
205-934-5077
205-975-7428 (fax)

Arizona

Arizona Cancer Center
University of Arizona
1515 North Campbell Avenue
Tucson, AZ 85724
520-626-2900
520-626-2284 (fax)

California

Jonsson Comprehensive
  Cancer Center
UCLA

Suite 1010
10920 Wilshire Boulevard
Los Angeles, CA 90024-6502
1-800-825-2631

Kenneth Norris, Jr.
  Comprehensive Cancer
  Center
University of Southern
  California
1441 Eastlake Avenue
Los Angeles, CA 90033-0800
1-800-522-6237
213-764-0816
213-764-3000 (fax)

Connecticut

Yale Cancer Center
Yale University School of
  Medicine
333 Cedar Street
New Haven, CT 06520-8028
203-785-4095
203-785-4116 (fax)

District of Columbia

Lombardi Cancer Research
  Center
Georgetown University
  Medical Center
3800 Reservoir Road N.W.
Washington, DC 20007
202-784-4000
202-687-6402 (fax)

Florida

Sylvester Comprehensive
  Cancer Center
University of Miami Medical
  School
1475 Northwest 12th Avenue
Miami, FL 33136
305-547-5757 or 1-800-432-0191

Maryland

The Johns Hopkins Oncology
  Center
601 North Caroline Street
Baltimore, MD 21287-0992
410-955-8964

Massachusetts

Dana-Farber Cancer Institute
44 Binney Street
Boston, MA 02115
617-632-3476

Michigan

Barbara Ann Karmanos
  Cancer Institute
Wayne State University

110 East Warren Avenue
Detroit, MI 48201-1379
313-745-4400
313-993-7165 (fax)

Comprehensive Cancer Center
University of Michigan
101 Simpson Drive
Ann Arbor, MI 48109-0752
313-936-9583 or 1-800-865-1125

New Hampshire

Norris Cotton Cancer Center
Dartmouth-Hitchcock Medical
  Center
One Medical Center Drive,
  Hinman Box 7920
Lebanon, NH 03756-0001
603-650-5527
603-650-4150 (fax)

New York

Kaplan Comprehensive Cancer
  Center
New York University Medical
  Center
550 First Avenue
New York, NY 10016
212-263-6485
212-263-8211 (fax)

Memorial Sloan-Kettering
  Cancer Center
1275 York Avenue

New York, NY 10021
212-639-6561 or 1-800-525-2225
212-717-3299 (fax)

Roswell Park Cancer Institute
Elm and Carlton Streets
Buffalo, NY 14263-0001
716-845-5772 or 1-800-767-9355
716-845-8261 (fax)

North Carolina

Comprehensive Cancer Center
Wake Forest University
Bowman Gray School of
  Medicine
Medical Center Boulevard
Winston-Salem, NC 27157-
  1082
919-716-2255
919-716-0293 (fax)

Duke Comprehensive Cancer
  Center
Duke University Medical
  Center
P.O. Box 3814
Durham, NC 27710
919-416-3843

Lineberger Comprehensive
  Cancer Center
University of North Carolina
School of Medicine, CB 7295
102 West Drive
Chapel Hill, NC 27599-7295
919-966-3036
919-966-3015 (fax)

Ohio

Comprehensive Cancer Center
Arthur G. James Cancer
  Hospital
Ohio State University
300 West 10th Avenue
Columbus, OH 43210-1240
614-293-5066 or 1-800-293-5066
614-293-3132 (fax)

Pennsylvania

Fox Chase Cancer Center
7701 Burholme Avenue
Philadelphia, PA 19111
215-728-2570
215-728-2571 (fax)

Pittsburgh Cancer Institute
Suite 405
Iroquois Building
3600 Forbes Avenue
Pittsburgh, PA 15213-3305
412-692-4670 or 1-800-237-4724
412-692-4665 (fax)

University of Pennsylvania
  Cancer Center
6th Floor
Penn Tower Hotel
3400 Spruce Street
Philadelphia, PA 19104-4383
215-662-6364 or 1-800-383-8722
215-346-5325 (fax)

Texas

M. D. Anderson Cancer
  Center
University of Texas
1515 Holcombe Boulevard
Houston, TX 77030
1-800-392-1611

San Antonio Cancer Institute
4450 Medical Drive
San Antonio, TX 78229
210-616-5798

Vermont

Vermont Regional Cancer
  Center
University of Vermont
1 South Prospect Street
Burlington, VT 05401-3498

802-656-4414
802-656-8788 (fax)

Washington

Fred Hutchinson Cancer
  Research Center
1124 Columbia Street
Seattle, WA 98104
206-667-5000
206-667-5268 (fax)

Wisconsin

Comprehensive Cancer Center
University of Wisconsin
600 Highland Avenue
Madison, WI 53792-0001
608-263-8090

CLINICAL CANCER CENTERS

There are seventeen National Cancer Institute–designated clinical
cancer centers, which conduct both basic and clinical research.
Clinical cancer centers have also been given thorough review by
the National Cancer Institute. Although they have not met all the
criteria to qualify as comprehensive centers, they qualify to provide investigational treatments.

California

City of Hope National Medical
  Center
Beckman Research Institute
1500 East Duarte Road
Duarte, CA 91010

818-301-8164 or 1-800-826-4673
818-930-5300 (fax)

Irvine Clinical Cancer Center
University of California at
  Irvine
101 The City Drive

Orange, CA 92668
714-456-8200
714-456-5039 (fax)

UCSD Cancer Center
University of California at San
    Diego
200 West Arbor Drive
San Diego, CA 92103-8421
619-543-3456
619-543-2639 (fax)

Colorado

University of Colorado Cancer
    Center
4200 East 9th Avenue,
    Box B188
Denver, CO 80262
1-800-473-2288
303-270-3304 (fax)

Illinois

Robert H. Lurie Cancer
    Center
Northwestern University
303 East Chicago Avenue
Chicago, IL 60611
312-908-5250
312-908-1372 (fax)

Cancer Research Center
University of Chicago
5841 South Maryland Avenue
Chicago, IL 60637-1470

312-702-9200 or 1-800-289-6333
312-702-9311 (fax)

Minnesota

Mayo Comprehensive Cancer
    Center
200 First Street S.W.
Rochester, MI 55905
507-284-4137
507-284-9349 (fax)

New York

Cancer Research Center
Albert Einstein College of
    Medicine
Montefiore Medical Center,
    Department of Oncology
111 East 210th Street
Bronx, NY 10467
718-920-4826

Columbia-Presbyterian Cancer
    Center
6th Floor, Room 435
Milstein Hospital Building
177 Fort Washington Avenue
New York, NY 10032
212-305-8610

University of Rochester Cancer
    Center
601 Elmwood Avenue,
    Box 704
Rochester, NY 14642
716-275-4911 or 1-800-462-6763

Ohio

Ireland Cancer Center
  at Case Western Reserve
  University
11100 Euclid Ave,
Cleveland, OH 44106-5065
216-844-5432

Pennsylvania

The Jefferson Cancer Center
Thomas Jefferson University
College Building, Suite 1014
1025 Walnut Street
Philadelphia, PA 19107-5799
1-800-426-3895

Tennessee

St. Jude Children's Research
  Hospital
332 North Lauderdale Street
Memphis, TN 38105-0318
901-495-3300

Vanderbilt Cancer Center
Vanderbilt University
649 Medical Research
  Building II

Nashville, TN 37232-6838
615-936-1782 or 1-800-811-8480

Utah

Huntsman Cancer Institute
University of Utah
50 North Medical Drive
Salt Lake City, UT 84112
1-800-488-2422

Virginia

Cancer Center
University of Virginia
Health Sciences Center
Hospital Box 334
Charlottesville, VA 22908
804-982-4190
804-982-0918 (fax)

Massey Cancer Center
Medical College of Virginia
P.O. Box 980037
401 College Street
Richmond, VA 23298-0037
804-828-5116

Consortium Cancer Center

The consortium cancer center works with state and local public
health departments to provide effective prevention and control
techniques learned from its research findings to those institutions
responsible for implementing populationwide public health programs. The center is heavily engaged in collaborations with insti-

tutions that conduct clinical trials to investigate new treatments and to coordinate community hospitals into a network of cooperating institutions in these research efforts.

Tennessee

Drew-Meharry-Morehouse Consortium Cancer Center
1005 D.B. Todd Boulevard
Nashville, TN 37208
615-327-6315
615-327-5838 (fax)

BASIC SCIENCE CANCER CENTERS

Basic science cancer centers engage almost entirely in basic research. However, some centers collaborate with outside clinical research investigators and with industry to generate medical applications from new discoveries in the laboratory. These centers are located as follows:

California

Armand Hammer Center for
   Cancer Biology
San Diego, CA

La Jolla Cancer Research
   Foundation
La Jolla, CA

Indiana

Purdue University Cancer
   Center
West Lafayette, IN

Maine

The Jackson Laboratory
Bar Harbor, ME

Massachusetts

Center for Cancer Research
Massachusetts Institute of
   Technology
Cambridge, MA

Nebraska

Eppley Institute
University of Nebraska
   Medical Center
Omaha, NE

New York

American Health Foundation
New York, NY

Cold Spring Harbor
    Laboratory
Cold Spring Harbor, NY

Pennsylvania

Wistar Institute Cancer Center
Philadelphia, PA

Wisconsin

McArdle Laboratory for
    Cancer Research
University of Wisconsin
Madison, WI

NIH CLINICAL CENTER

Warren Grant Magnuson Clinical Center

The National Institutes of Health has a medical research center and hospital—the Warren Grant Magnuson Clinical Center, located in Bethesda, Maryland, just outside of Washington, D.C. The hospital portion of the Clinical Center, with room for 540 patients, is especially designed for medical research. The number of beds available for a particular project and the length of the waiting list of qualified patients are important in determining whether and when you can be admitted. Research on a particular disease may allow only one or two patients to be studied at any given time. The Clinical Center provides nursing and medical care without charge for patients who are being studied in clinical research program.

You can be treated at the Clinical Center only if your case fits into a research project. Each project is designed to answer scientific questions and has specific medical eligibility requirements. For this reason you must be referred by your own doctor, who can supply the Clinical Center with the needed medical information, such as your diagnosis and details of your medical history. If your doctor feels that you might benefit by participating in a cancer research study at NIH, the doctor should call the National Cancer Institute's Public Inquiries Office at 301-496-5583 or write to the Clinical Director, National Cancer Institute, Building 10, Room 12N214, Bethesda, MD 20892.

HOSPITALS THAT PROVIDE CRYOSURGERY

Because cryosurgery is a relatively new treatment for prostate cancer, not all hospitals are using this treatment. The following hospitals presently use cryosurgery for treatment of prostate cancer.

Alabama

Springhill Memorial Hospital
Mobile, AL

University of Alabama Hospital
Birmingham, AL

California

Alhambra Hospital
Arcadia, CA

Century City Hospital
Los Angeles, CA

John Wayne Cancer Institute
(St. John's Hospital)
Santa Monica, CA

Long Beach Memorial
Long Beach, CA

Sherman Oaks Hospital
Sherman Oaks, CA

Sutter Memorial Hospital
Sacramento, CA

UCI Medical Center
Irvine, CA

UCLA Medical Center
Los Angeles, CA

UCSD Medical Center,
   Hillcrest
San Diego, CA

UCSF Medical Center
San Francisco, CA

VA Medical Center
San Francisco, CA

Colorado

North Suburban Medical
   Center
Thronton, CO

Radiology Imaging Association
Englewood, CO

University Hospital
Denver, CO

Connecticut

Yale-New Haven Hospital
New Haven, CT

Delaware

St. Francis Hospital
Wilmington, DE

District of Columbia

Walter Reed Army Medical
  Center
Washington, D.C.

Washington Hospital Center
Washington, D.C.

Florida

Boca Raton Community
  Hospital
Boca Raton, FL

Cleveland Clinic Hospital
Ft. Lauderdale, FL

H. Lee Moffitt Cancer Center
Tampa, FL

Jupiter Medical Center
Jupiter, FL

Lee Memorial Hospital
Fort Myers, FL

MD Anderson Cancer Center
Orlando Regional Medical
  Center
Orlando, FL

Mount Sinai Medical Center
Miami Beach, FL

Palms of Pasadena Hospital
St. Petersburg, FL

Princeton Hospital
Orlando, FL

Shands Hospital
University of Florida
Gainesville, FL

South Miami Hospital
South Miami, FL

St. Luke's Hospital of the
  Mayo Clinic
Jacksonville, FL

St. Vincent's Medical Center
Jacksonville, FL

Georgia

Crawford Long Hospital of
  Emory University
Atlanta, GA

Emory University Hospital
Atlanta, GA

Georgia Baptist Medical
  Center
Atlanta, GA

Illinois

Loyola University Medical
  Center
Chicago, IL

Rush Presbyterian-St. Luke's
  Medical Center
Chicago, IL

Swedish Covenant Hospital
Chicago, IL

University of Chicago Hospital
Chicago, IL

Weiss Memorial Hospital
Chicago, IL

Indiana

Methodist Hospital of Indiana
Indianapolis, IN

Northeast Indiana Urology
Fort Wayne, IN

St. Vincent Hospital
Indianapolis, IN

Welborn Memorial Baptist
Hospital
Evansville, IN

Kentucky

Alliant Medical Pavilion
Louisville, KY

Louisiana

Doctor's Hospital
Metairie, LA

Meadowcrest Hospital
Gretna, LA

Tulane University Hospital
and Clinic
New Orleans, LA

Maryland

St. Agnes Hospital
Baltimore, MD

University of Maryland
Baltimore, MD

Massachusetts

Boston University Medical
Center
Boston, MA

Metrowest Medical Center
Framingham, MA

New England Medical Center
Boston, MA

University of Massachusetts
Medical Center
Worcester, MA

Michigan

Bon Secours Hospital
Grosse Point, MI

Catherine McAuley Health
System
Ann Arbor, MI

Crittenton Hospital
Rochester, MI

Harper Hospital
Detroit, MI

McLaren Regional Medical
Center
Flint, MI

Metropolitan Hospital
Grand Rapids, MI

St. John Hospital
Detroit, MI

University of Michigan
Medical Center
Ann Arbor, MI

William Beaumont Hospital
Royal Oak, MI

Minnesota

Lake Region Hospital
Fergus Falls, MN

Missouri

Boone Hospital Center
Columbia, MO

Cox Medical Center
Springfield, MO

St. Anthony's Medical Center
St. Louis, MO

St. Luke's Hospital
Kansas City, MO

Nebraska

University of Nebraska
  Medical Center
Omaha, NE

New Jersey

Hackensack Medical Center
Hackensack, NJ

Robert Wood Johnson
  Hospital
New Brunswick, NJ

Underwood Memorial
  Hospital
Woodbury, NJ

New York

Albany Medical Center
  Hospital
Albany, NY

Albany Memorial Hospital
Albany, NY

Beth Israel Medical Center
New York, NY

Brooklyn Hospital Center
Brooklyn, NY

Genesee Hospital
Rochester, NY

Jamaica Medical Center
Jamaica, NY

Long Island College Hospital
Brooklyn, NY

Memorial Sloan Kettering
  Cancer Center
New York, NY

New York Hospital
New York, NY

Presbyterian Hospital
New York, NY

Roswell Park Cancer Institute
Buffalo, NY

Staten Island University
  Hospital
Staten Island, NY

University Medical Center
Stony Brook, NY

Victory Memorial Hospital
Brooklyn, NY

North Carolina

Pitt County Memorial Hospital
Greenville, NC

Ohio

Bethesda Oak Hospital
Cincinnati, OH

Case Western Reserve
University Hospital
Cleveland, OH

Cleveland Clinic Hospital
Cleveland, OH

Meridia Hillcrest Hospital
Mayfield Heights, OH

Medical College of Ohio
Hospital
Toledo, OH

Ohio State University Hospital
Columbus, OH

Park Medical Center
Columbus, OH

Parma Community General
Hospital
Parma, OH

St. Elizabeth Medical Center
Tulsa, OH

Oklahoma

St. John Medical Center
Tulsa, OK

Pennsylvania

Allegheny General Hospital
Pittsburgh, PA

Bryn Mawr Hospital
Bryn Mawr, PA

Pennsylvania Hospital
Philadelphia, PA

Phoenixville Hospital
Phoenixville, PA

Presbyterian University
Medical Center
Pittsburgh, PA

Temple University Hospital
Philadelphia, PA

Thomas Jefferson University
Hospital
Philadelphia, PA

University of Pennsylvania
Medical Center
Philadelphia, PA

South Carolina

MUSC Medical Center
Charleston, SC

Roper Hospital
Charleston, SC

Spartanburg Regional Medical
Center
Spartanburg, SC

Tennessee

Baptist Memorial Hospital
Memphis, TN

Jackson-Madison County
General Hospital
Jackson, TN

UT Bowld Hospital
Memphis, TN

Texas

Lubbock Methodist Hospital
Lubbock, TX

M.D. Anderson Cancer Center
Houston, TX

Medical City Dallas Hospital
Dallas, TX

Providence Health Center
Waco, TX

Scott and White Memorial
Hospital
Temple, TX

Spring Branch Medical Center
Houston, TX

University of Texas Medical
Branch
Galveston, TX

Utah

University of Utah Hospital
and Clinics
Salt Lake City, UT

Virginia

University of Virginia Health
Science Center
Charlottesville, VA

Washington

University of Washington
Medical Center
Seattle, WA

West Virginia

Charleston Area Medical
Center
Charleston, WV

Wisconsin

Meriter Hospital
Madison, WI

St. Francis Hospital
Milwaukee, WI

St. Luke's Medical Center/
Aurora Health Care
Milwaukee, WI

University of Wisconsin
Hospital and Clinics
Madison, WI

International

Academic Hospital
Middelheim
Antwerpen, Belgium

Center of Urological
Ultrasound
Trieste, Italy

Chang Gung Memorial
Hospital
Taipei, Taiwan

Herlev Hospital
Herlev, Denmark

Johannes Gutenberg
Universität
Mainz, Germany

Medizinische Enrichtungen
der Universität zu Köln
Köln, Germany

Östra Hospital
Göteborg, Sweden

Tom Baker Cancer Center
Calgary, Alberta, Canada

University Hospital Nejmegen
Nejmegen, Netherlands

NATIONWIDE DIRECT-HELP SERVICES AND ORGANIZATIONS

American Association of Sex Educators, Counselors and Therapists (ASECT)
Suite 1717
435 North Michigan Avenue
Chicago, IL 60611
312-644-0828
Provides names of sex therapists in your area.

American Foundation for Urologic Disease
300 West Pratt Street, Suite 401
Baltimore, MD 21201-2463
800-828-7866
Provides educational opportunities for the public, patients, and health care professionals about urologic diseases. Support groups: Us Too, Bladder Health Council, and Prostate Cancer Survivors Network.

CAN ACT (Cancer Patients Action Alliance)
26 College Place
Brooklyn, NY 11201
718-522-4607
Addresses problems of access to advanced cancer treatments, barriers created by the Food and Drug Administration's drug approval process, and restrictive insurance reimbursement policies.

Cancer Care, Inc., and National Cancer Care Foundation
1180 Avenue of the Americas
New York, NY 10036
212-221-3300
A nonprofit social service agency helping patients and families cope with emotional, financial, and psychological consequences of cancer. Provides free individual, family, and group counseling. Financial counseling is also available as is financial assistance for home care and transportation.

Cancer Conquerors Foundation
P.O. Box 3444
Fullerton, CA 92634
800-238-6479
Offers cancer survival training programs and self-study materials
with specific emphasis on body/mind/spirit.

Cancer Information Service
1-800-4-CANCER (1-800-422-6237)
Nationwide telephone service, a program of the National Cancer
Institute, for cancer patients and their families, the public, and
health care professionals. Cancer Information Service information specialists have extensive training in providing up-to-date and
understandable information about cancer. They can answer questions in English and Spanish and send free printed material. Cancer Information Service offices serve specific geographic areas and
have information about cancer-related services and resources in
their region.

CaP CURE
The Association for the Cure of Cancer of the Prostate
1250 Fourth Street, Suite 360
Santa Monica, CA 90401
310-458-2873
Dedicated to finding a cure for prostate cancer by funding cancer
research. Funds Prostate Cancer Genetic Research Study.

Clinical Center of the National Institutes of Health (Warren
Grant Magnuson Clinical Center)
Patient Referral Service
Building 10, Room IC 255
9000 Rockville Pike
Bethesda, Maryland
301-496-4891

Choice in Dying
(formerly Concern for Dying & Society for the Right to Die)
200 Varick Street

New York, NY 10014-4810
800-989-WILL
Provides the latest information on the right to die, living wills,
and so on.

Corporate Angel Network, Inc.
Westchester County Airport, Building 1
White Plains, NY 10604
914-328-1313
800-328-4226 (fax)
This service uses available space on corporate airplanes for trans-
porting cancer patients in need of transportation to treatment
centers.

Families Against Cancer (FACT)
P.O. Box 588
Dewitt, NY 13214
315-446-5326
Grassroots coalition of cancer patients, families, and friends seek-
ing new and more vigorous national policy on cancer.

Help for Incontinent People
P.O. Box 544
Union, South Carolina 29379
800-BLADDER
Information on the benefits and drawbacks of various treatments
for incontinence. Maintains referral service of doctors and therapists who treat incontinence.

Hereditary Cancer Institute
Creighton University
Omaha, NE 68178
402-280-1746
Nonprofit organization devoted to the study of the genetics of
familial cancer. Maintains a registry of families interested in participating in its work.

Hospice
See *National Hospice Organization.*

I Can Cope
American Cancer Society
1-800-ACS-2345
A patient education program of the American Cancer Society designed to help patients, families, and friends cope with the day-to-day issues of living with cancer. Look in the telephone directory white pages for your local American Cancer Society chapter.

Impotence Institute of America, Inc.
2020 Pennsylvania Avenue NW, Suite 292
Washington, DC 20006
800-669-1630
Provides information on impotence and its treatment.

Joint Commission on Accreditation of Healthcare Organizations (JCAHO)
1 Renaissance Boulevard
Oak Brook Terrace, IL 60181
708-916-5800
Hospital accrediting organization. Will tell you if hospital has been accredited by JCAHO.

Lymphedema Network
See *National Lymphedema Network.*

Man to Man
910 Contento Street
Sarasota, FL 34242
812-355-4987
A national support network for prostate cancer survivors. Contact them or the American Cancer Society for the chapter nearest you.

National Association of Oncology Social Workers
1275 York Avenue, MRI 1107
New York, NY 10021
212-639-7015
National association of professional social workers in cancer.

National Coalition for Cancer Survivorship
1010 Wayne Avenue, 5th Floor
Silver Spring, MD 20910
301-650-8868
Network of groups and individuals offering information and support to cancer survivors and families. Holds annual conference on survivor issues. Publishes *Networker* magazine and maintains national database.

National Consumers League
815 15th Street, NW, Suite 92N
Washington, DC 20005
202-639-8140
National nonprofit membership organization offering publications on a range of health issues such as hospice, home health care, and insurance.

National Council Against Health Fraud
Consumer Health Information Research Institute
3521 Broadway
Kansas City, MO 04111
1-800-821-6671
Provides information on questionable health practices and organizations.

National Hospice Organization
1901 North Moore Street, Suite 901
Arlington, VA 22209
703-243-5900 (publication line)
1-800-658-8898
An association of groups that provide hospice care. Designed to promote and maintain hospice care and to encourage support for patients and family members.

National Lymphedema Network
2211 Post Street, Suite 404
San Francisco, CA 94115
1-800-541-3259
Nonprofit network provides printed information and other assis-

tance to those who develop lymphedema as a result of lymph node surgery or radiation therapy. Serves as a resource center for patients and health care professionals, and publishes a newsletter.

National Society of Genetic Counselors
233 Canterbury Drive
Wallingford, PA 19086-6617
610-872-7608
Answers questions about genetic counseling. Can provide a list of genetic counselors specializing in cancer.

Office of Alternative Medicine
National Institutes of Health
Building 31, Room B1C35
Bethesda, MD 20892
Funds research on alternative treatments. University of Texas Health Science Center in Houston has been granted award for research in cancer.

PAACT
See *Patient Advocates for Advanced Cancer Treatments*.

Patient Advocates for Advanced Cancer Treatments (PAACT)
P.O. Box 141695
Grand Rapids, MI 49514-1695
616-453-1744
616-453-1846 (fax)
Provides information on treatments for prostate cancer. Concentrates mainly on nonsurgical treatments.

PDQ (Protocol Data Query)
1-800-4-CANCER
National Cancer Institute's computerized listing of up-to-date information for patients and health professionals on latest cancer treatments, research studies, clinical trials, promising cancer treatments, and organizations and doctors involved with cancer. Patient component available through phone number listed. Physicians may use an office computer or medical library services to obtain professional information.

Prostate Cancer Genetic Research Study
Fred Hutchinson Cancer Research Center
1124 Columbia Street, MP381
Seattle, WA 98104
1-800-777-3035
Nationwide research project exploring why some families have
several male relatives with prostate cancer.

Prostate Cancer Support Network
300 West Pratt Street, Suite 401
Baltimore, MD 21201
1-800-248-7866
Nationwide network of prostate support groups.

R.A. Bloch Cancer Foundation, Inc.
The Cancer Hotline
4410 Main Street
Kansas City, MO 64111
816-932-8453
Provides information for people diagnosed with cancer to help
locate best treatments.

Sex Information and Education Council of U.S.
130 West 42nd Street
New York, NY 10036
Provides information on sexuality and illness.

(The) Simon Foundation for Continence
Box 815
Wilmette, IL 60091
1-800-23-SIMON
Provides information on the management and treatment of in-
continence.

US–TOO INTERNATIONAL
930 North York Road, Suite 50
Hinsdale, IL 60521-2993
708-323-1002
708-323-1003

A national support network for prostate cancer survivors. Contact them for the chapter nearest you.

(The) Wellness Community
2716 Ocean Park Boulevard, Suite 1040
Santa Monica, CA 90404-5211
310-453-2300
Provides free psychosocial support to people fighting to recover from cancer as an adjunct to conventional medical treatment. Has 14 facilities throughout the nation.

DATABASE SOURCES AND PUBLICATIONS

There has been an explosion of information about every aspect of cancer. It is suggested that you use the sources listed as a starting point and guide in your search for information.

DATABASES

Electronic information services have become a convenient, cost-effective method of accessing information by computer. Most hospital and university libraries subscribe to specific on-line databases, or they can be accessed from personal computers via a modem.

INTERNET

The Internet is a large "network of networks" in which regional nets are interconnected, communicating a wide variety of information at amazing speed. You can access the Internet through your personal computer, through special software, such as Gopher or Netscape, or with one of the major on-line services—CompuServe, Prodigy, and America Online. There are forums, chat areas, on-line medical clinics, bulletin boards, and message boards. Some of the information is quite useful and from very legitimate, authorized sources (both the National Cancer Institute and the American Cancer Society have information on-line). You need to understand that there are no built-in controls or restrictions to regulate the kind of information that is being given. Some of the information on-line is from marketing and selling enterprises trying to get you to buy their products. Others are patients who are sharing their experiences. Be sure you look at the source of what is being presented. Most on-line services tell you that you are taking the advice at your own risk. Here are some addresses to start with in accessing the World Wide Web:

- **National Cancer Institute, including PDQ**: http://wwwi-cic.nci.nih.gov/
- **American Cancer Society**: http://www.cancer.org
- **Prostate Cancer Home Page**: http://www.cancer.med.umich.edu/prostcan/prostcan.html
- **Prostate Cancer Infoline**: http://www.comed.com/Prostate

CancerFax
National Cancer Institute
Bethesda, MD 20892
301-402-5874
301-402-7403 (for technical assistance)
This is a quick and easy way to obtain cancer information from the National Cancer Institute by calling the CancerFax computer from your fax machine. It operates 24 hours a day, seven days a week, with no charge other than a telephone call from your fax machine to the CancerFax computer in Bethesda, Maryland. You can request information statements in English or Spanish from the National Cancer Institute's PDQ System as well as fact sheets on various cancer topics from the National Cancer Institute's Office of Cancer Communications.

International Cancer Information Center
National Cancer Institute
Building 82, Room 107
Bethesda, MD 20892
301-402-5874
Collects, updates, and maintains the following databases, which are specifically cancer related:

- The PDQ database, which contains the latest updated information concerning cancer treatment and clinical trials, is available on-line through the National Library of Medicine's MEDLARS system. The National Cancer Institute is responsible for licensing PDQ to hospitals, universities, and other nonprofit institutions.

- The Cancerlit database, which contains the majority of cancer-related citations from MEDLINE, supplemented with additional citations of books, meeting abstracts, theses, and other publications.
- CancerFax, which makes treatment, supportive care, and cancer screening statements from PDQ available via fax in either English or Spanish. Statements are available for health professionals as well as for the general public.
- CancerNet, which makes treatment, supportive care, and cancer screening statements from PDQ available via electronic mail.

National Library of Medicine
8600 Rockville Pike
Bethesda, MD 20894
301-496-6193
1-800-638-8480
The National Library of Medicine's MEDLARS is a 24-hour-a-day system that allows for cost-effective searching of specialized databases. Its specific databases include

- MEDLINE (abstracts to journal articles).
- CATLINE (records of books).
- AVLINE (records of audiovisuals).
- CHEMLINE (information about chemical substances).
- HEALTH (information about health care services).
- TOXLINE (toxicological information).
- DIRLINE (directory of 15,000 information resources).
- AIDLINE (AIDS-related references).
- PDQ (advances in cancer treatment and clinical trials).

The GRATEFUL MED database allows for easy access to the National Library of Medicine's vast collection of medical and health science information. An average search costs about $3.00.

HEALTH SCIENCES JOURNALS

The *Index Medicus*, which is found in medical libraries, most university and college libraries, and some public libraries, lists articles appearing in over 2,400 health sciences journals. There are also dozens of oncology-related journals and bibliographic resource books. The resource *Medical Health Books and Serials* is available in most medical libraries.

NONTECHNICAL MAGAZINES

Articles that appear in the most popular nontechnical magazines and journals are listed in *The Reader's Guide to Periodical Literature* or in *The Public Affairs Information Service.* These two guides are usually available either in book or electronic form in most public libraries. Look in the index under the subject in which you are interested or, if you know it, under the author's name.

MONEY MATTERS

Cancer can impose heavy economic burdens on both patients and their families. For many people, a portion of medical expenses is paid by their health insurance plan. An employer's personnel office or an insurance company can provide information about the types of medical costs covered by a particular policy. Medical costs that are not covered by insurance policies sometimes can be deducted from your annual income before taxes.

For individuals who do not have health insurance or who need additional financial assistance, several resources are available, including government-sponsored programs and services supported by voluntary organizations.

Before leaving the hospital, discuss any concerns you may have about medical costs with a hospital social worker or patient accounts representative. They often can help patients identify appropriate sources of aid and can also help patients negotiate a payment plan with which the patient feels comfortable.

- Medicare, a health insurance program that is administered by the Social Security Administration, is designed for people over 65 or those who are permanently disabled. The telephone number of the closest Social Security office is listed in the telephone directory or can be obtained by calling 1-800-772-1213.

- Medicaid is a program for people who need financial assistance for medical expenses. It is coordinated by the Health Care Financing Administration of the Department of Health and Human Services and is administered by individual states. Information about coverage is available from a hospital social worker or a local public health or social services office.

- The federal government also administers the Hill–Burton Program, through which many medical facilities and hospitals provide free or low-cost care. Hill–Burton hospitals receive government construction and modernization funds and are required by law to provide some services to people who cannot afford to pay. For eligibility information call 1-800-638-0742.

- If a cancer patient or his or her spouse is or has been a member of the armed forces, the U.S. Department of Veterans Affairs (VA) may be able to help with health care costs. The VA provides hospital care covering the full range of medical services. Treatment is available for all service-related conditions and some nonservice-related ones. For questions about veterans' benefits, call 1-800-827-1000.

- The Civilian Health and Medical Program of the VA is a medical benefits program for dependents of veterans through which the VA provides payment for medical services and supplies obtained from civilian sources. Any VA health care facility can provide information about these programs.

- The federal government's Civilian Health and Medical Programs of the Uniformed Services (CHAMPUS) helps pay for civilian medical care for spouses and children of active-duty Uniformed Services personnel, retired Uniformed Services personnel and their spouses and children, and spouses and children of active-duty or retired active-duty personnel who have died. CHAMPUS will pay for treatment for cancer patients on clinical trials (see Chapter 14). Information about CHAMPUS is available from the CHAMPUS Advisor/Health

Benefits Advisor at your nearest Uniformed Services medical facility or write to Information Office of CHAMPUS, Aurora, CO 80045.

- The American Cancer Society offers counseling, transportation, and rehabilitation programs. Consult your telephone directory for your local office.
- Groups such as the Salvation Army, United Way, Lutheran Social Services, Jewish Social Services, the Lions Club, Associated Catholic Charities, as well as churches and synagogues sometimes provide financial help.

American Association of Retired Persons (AARP)
601 E Street, N.W.
Washington, DC 20049
202-443-2277
1-800-456-2277 (pharmacy service price quote)
Provides legislative advocacy, programs such as Medicare/Medicaid assistance, and the Breast Cancer and Mammography Awareness information campaign for people 50 or older. Wide range of membership benefits include *Modern Maturity* magazine and Medicare supplementary insurance. Will quote prices for prescription medications on toll-free number.

Blue Cross and Blue Shield Association
676 North St. Clair Street
Chicago, Illinois 60601
312-440-6000
Provides information on Blue Cross/Blue Shield coverage offered in every state, including the availability of annual open enrollment periods.

Disabled American Veterans
807 Main Avenue, S.W.
Washington, DC 20024
202-554-3501
A national organization serving veterans and their dependents. Approximately 3,000 chapters offer counseling, educational materials, support groups, transportation, conferences, and a newsletter.

Health Insurance Association of America (HIAA)
1025 Connecticut Avenue, N.E., Suite 1200
Washington, DC 20036
202-223-7808
A trade association representing major health insurance companies. Offers consumer publications about health insurance,
long-term care insurance, and Medicare supplement insurance.

Medical Information Bureau Inc. (MIB)
P.O. Box 105
Esses Station
Boston, MA 02112
617-426-3660
MIB can send a copy of your medical records so that you can
verify the information in them and correct any inaccuracies. Call
MIB first to find out the type of information it requires to process
your request.

The National Insurance Consumer Helpline
1-800-942-4242
Provides information on all types of insurance. A joint project of
the American Council on Life Insurance, the Health Insurance
Association of America, and the Insurance Information Institute.

Pension and Welfare Benefits Administration
U.S. Department of Labor, Room N-5669
200 Constitution Avenue, N.W.
Washington, DC 20210
202-523-8521
Enforces your rights under COBRA to continued health insurance
coverage and provides information about how to enforce your
rights to equal job benefits under ERISA.

U.S. Department of Health and Human Services
Social Security Administration
Baltimore, MD 21235
1-800-772-1213
Provides information on Medicare.

HEALTH COVERAGE FOR THE HARD-TO-INSURE

A number of states currently sell comprehensive health insurance to state residents with serious medical conditions who are unable to find a company to insure them. Contact your state Department of Insurance to find out whether your state has such a program or what assistance the department can offer you.

Bibliography

Among the many resources used in completing this book, we found these particularly useful:

Albertson, Peter. Clinical crossroads. *JAMA* 274:1, 1995.

Bolger JJ, et al. Strontium-89 (Metastron) versus external beam radiotherapy in patients with painful bone metastases secondary to prostatic cancer: Preliminary report of a multicenter trial. *Seminars in Oncology* 20:3, 1993.

Brody J. Personal Health: Impotence. *New York Times*, August 9, 1995.

Brown ML, Fireman B. Evaluation of direct medical costs related to cancer, *Journal of the National Cancer Institute* 87:6, 1995.

Catalona WJ, Basler JW. Return of erections and urinary continence following nerve sparing radical retropubic prostatectomy. *Journal of Urology* 150:3, 1993.

Chen YT, et al. Using proportions of free to total prostate-specific antigen, age and total prostate-specific antigen to predict the probability of prostate cancer. *Urology* 47:518–24, 1996.

Chodak GW, et al. Results of conservative management of clinically localized prostate cancer. *New England Journal of Medicine* 330: 4, 1994.

Crawford, ED, et al. A controlled trial of leuprolide with and without flutamide in prostatic carcinoma. *New England Journal of Medicine* 327:7, 1992.

D'Amico AV, Coleman CN. Role of interstitial radiotherapy in the management of clinically organ-confined prostate cancer: the jury is still out. *Journal of Clinical Oncology* 14:304–315, 1996.

Das S, Crawford ED. *Cancer of the Prostate.* Marcel Dekker, 1993.

DeVita VT, Hellman S, Rosenberg SA. *Cancer: Principles and practice of oncology.* J.B. Lippincott, 1993.

Eisner E, Tobin E. "What Should We Tell Men about Prostate Cancer," Focus Group Research, National Cancer Institute, October 1992.

Fracchia JA. Prostate cancer: Why all the current interest? *Primary Care and Cancer* 13:2, 1993.

Graversen PH, et al. Radical prostatectomy versus expectant primary treatment in stages I and II prostatic cancer: A fifteen-year follow-up. *Urology* 36:6, 1990.

Greskovich FJ, et al. Complications following external beam radiation therapy for prostate cancer: An analysis of patients treated with and without staging pelvic lymphadenectomy. *Journal of Urology* 146:3, 1991.

Gromley GJ, et al. The effect of finasteride in men with benign prostatic hyperplasia, *New England Journal of Medicine*, 327:17, 1992.

Laramore GE, et al. Fast neutron radiotherapy in the treatment for locally advanced prostate cancer. Final report of a radiation therapy oncology group randomized clinical trial. *American Journal of Clinical Oncology* 16:2, 1993.

Linet OI, et al. Efficacy and safety of intracavernosal alprostadil in men with erectile dysfunction. *New England Journal of Medicine* 334:873–87, 1996.

Lu-Yao GL, et al. An assessment of radical prostatectomy: Time trends, geographic variation and outcomes. *JAMA* 269:20, 1993.

Lu-Yao GL, et al. Follow up prostate cancer treatments after radical prostatectomy: A population-based study. *Journal of the National Cancer Institute* 88:166–73, 1996.

Miller, RJ, et al. Percutaneous transperineal cryosurgery of the prostate as salvage treatment for post radiation recurrence of adenocarcinoma. *Cancer* 77:1510–14, 1196.

Murphy GP, et al. *American Cancer Society Textbook of Clinical Oncology.* American Cancer Society, 1995.

National Cancer Institute Budget, 1996, pp. 325–346, National Institutes of Health, 1995.

National Cancer Institute. *PDQ Prostate Cancer State-of-the-Art Treatment Summary and PDQ Prostate Cancer Clinical Trials.* June 1996.

National Cancer Institute. *What You Need to Know about Cancer of the Prostate.* National Institutes of Health, 1992.

National Institutes of Health. *Alternative Medicine: Expanding Medical Horizons.* National Institutes of Health, 1995.

National Institutes of Health. National Institute of Health Consensus Development Conference statement: The management of clinically localized prostate cancer. *JAMA* 258:19, 1987.

Porter AT, et al. Brachytherapy for prostate cancer. *CA: A Journal for Clinicians* 45:3, 1995.

Schultz P, Scher HI. *Primary Care & Cancer* 13:2, 1993.

Tchetgen MB, et al. Ejaculation increases the serum prostate-specific antigen concentration. *Urology* 47:511–516, 1996.

Walsh PC. Radical prostatectomy. *Campbell's Urology,* 5th ed. W.B. Saunders, 1995.

Walsh PC, Worthington JF. *The prostate: a guide for men and the women who love them.* The Johns Hopkins University Press, 1995.

Wasson JH, et al. A structured literature review of treatment for localized prostate cancer. *Archives of Family Medicine* 2:487, 1993.

Woolf, SH. Screening for prostate cancer with prostate-specific antigen. *The New England Journal of Medicine* 333:21, 1995.

Zincke H, et al. Radical prostatectomy for clinically localized prostate cancer, long-term results of 1,143 patients from a single institution. *Journal of Clinical Oncology* 12:11, 1991.

About the Authors

MARION MORRA is the Associate Director of the Yale Cancer Center in New Haven, Connecticut. She is Associate Research Scientist at the Yale School of Medicine and Associate Clinical Professor at the Yale School of Nursing. Marion is widely published, having written articles and authored books for both health professionals and the public, with emphasis on health, especially in the field of cancer. She serves on major national committees for the National Cancer Institute and the American Cancer Society.

EVE POTTS has been writing on medical subjects for more than 30 years. Her expertise is in making difficult medical information easy to understand. She has served as a medical writer and consultant to the Department of Health and Human Services and many medically oriented companies and institutions. Her interest in history is represented by another book, *Westport, A Special Place, 1987.*

The two authors, who are sisters, have collaborated on five other books: three editions of the best-selling book for cancer patients *Choices* (Avon Books, 1980, 1987, and 1994), *Triumph: Getting Back to Normal When You Have Cancer* (Avon Books, 1990), and *Understanding Your Immune System* (1986). In 1993, the authors received the Natalie Davis Springarn Writer's Award from the National Coalition for Cancer Survivors for "their valuable contributions to the literature of survivorship and for their books, *Choices* and *Triumph.*" They also were awarded the 1995 National Health Information Silver Award, which honors the nation's best consumer health information programs and materials, for *Choices.*

244 ABOUT THE AUTHORS

In the process of reading and using this book, questions that are not included in it may come to your mind. The authors would be pleased if you would share your thoughts with them. Kindly send any comments to:

Eve Potts, Marion Morra
c/o Avon Books
1350 Avenue of the Americas
New York, New York 10019

Index

A

AARP. *See* American Association of Retired Persons

Acid phosphatase, 16

Active surveillance. *See* Watchful waiting

Adenocarcinomas, 52

Alprostadil (Caverject), 189

Alternative treatments. *See* Unproven treatments

American Association of Retired Persons (AARP), 236

American Association of Sex Educators, Counselors and Therapists (ASECT), 183, 224

American Board of Certified Specialties, 79

American Board of Medical Specialties, 200

American Cancer Society, 199, 200, 203

division offices, 204–8

national office, 204

programs, 198–99, 227, 236

American Foundation for Urologic Disease, 224

American Urological Association, 199

Anesthesia, 97–98

coming out of, 100–1

epidural, 97

general, 97

questions to ask concerning, 98

spinal, 97

Anesthesiologists, 98

Antiandrogens, 154

ASECT. *See* American Association of Sex Educators, Counselors and Therapists

Associated Catholic Charities, 236

245

External radiation. *See*
  Radiation treatment

F

Families Against Cancer
  (FACT), 226
Fat, in diet, 27
Financial matters, 234–38
Finasteride. *See* Proscar
Flutamide, 151
  side effects of, 151
Fractionation, 118
Free molecules, 10

G

Genes, prostate cancer, 27
Genetic research, 164
Gerson therapy, 176
Gleason grades, 50
  chart, 51
  determining, 50
  meaning of, 50
  treatment based on, 51
Grading systems, 50–52

H

Hair loss, radiation treatment
  and, 121–22
Health Insurance Association
  of America (HIAA), 237
Health maintenence
  organizations (HMOs):
  biopsies and, 41
  choosing doctor and, 30
  second opinions and, 84
Heavy-ion radiation,166–67
Hellman, Samuel, 113
Help for Incontinent People,
  196, 226
Hematopoietic growth
  factors. *See* Tumor
  growth factors
Hereditary Cancer Institute,
  226
Heredity, prostate cancer
  and, 26, 164
High-LET radiation, 166
Hill-Burton Program, 235
HMOs. *See* Health
  maintenence
  organizations
Hormone blockage, 166
Hormone treatment, 61, 64,
  75, 147–56
  antiandrogens, 150–51, 154
  before prostatectomy, 90
  before radiation seeding,
  129
  before external radiation,
  113
  for bone metastases, 155–
  56

L

Laetrile, 176–77
Laparoscopic lymph node
    dissection. *See* Lymph
    node dissection
Laparoscopic
    lymphadenectomy. *See*
    Lymph node dissection
Laser surgery, 65
LHRHs. *See* Luteinizing
    hormone-releasing
    hormone agonists
Linear accelerator, 112
Lions Club, 236
Livingston treatment, 178–79
Lupron, 149, 150
Luteinizing hormone-
    releasing hormone
    agonists (LHRHs), 149–
    50, 154
Lutheran Social Services, 236
Lymph node dissection
    (lymphadenectomy), 48,
    65, 94–96
  before radiation seeding,
    130–32
  before external radiation,
    113–14
  procedure, 114
  prostatectomy, 94–95
Lymphadenectomy. *See*
    Lymph node dissection
Lymphedema, 106–7, 114,
    121, 198
Lymphedema Network. *See*
    National Lymphedema
    Network

M

Macrobiotic diet, 175–76
Magnetic resonance imaging
    (MRI), 45, 47
  cost of, 47
  endorectal coil, 47–48
  procedure, 47
Man to Man, 199, 227
Margins, 28
Medicaid, 235
  radiation treatment and,
    125
*Medical Health Books and
    Serials,* 234
Medical Information Bureau,
    Inc. (MIB), 237
Medicare, 234–35
  billing balance and, 84–85
  cryosurgery and, 146
  radiation treatment and,
    125
  treatment costs and, 84–85
Medigap, 84
  radiation treatment and,
    125
Metabolic therapy, 176–77
Metastases, 29–30, 54–58
  bone, 155
  Strontium-89, 155–56
Metastron. *See* Strontium-89
Microwave 19, 34, 167
Mitomycin, 162
Mitoxantrone, 162
Monoclonal antibodies, 160
MRI. *See* Magnetic resonance
    imaging